Treatment Dilemmas for Vulnerable Patients in Oral Health

Treatment Dilemmas for Vulnerable Patients in Oral Health

Alexander Mersel

Editor

Treatment Dilemmas for Vulnerable Patients in Oral Health

Clinical and Ethical Issues

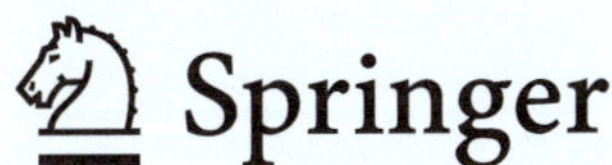

Springer

Editor
Alexander Mersel
Community Dentistry Hadassah School
of Dental Medicine
University of Jerusalem
Jerusalem, Israel

ISBN 978-3-031-08437-9   ISBN 978-3-031-08435-5   (eBook)
https://doi.org/10.1007/978-3-031-08435-5

This Springer imprint is published by the registered company Springer Nature Switzerland AG
The registered company address is: Gewerbestrasse 11, 6330 Cham, Switzerland

Foreword

As we embrace the twenty-first century reality of an ever-expanding global geriatric population, are we as dental professionals adequately prepared to successfully address the significant and oft-times challenging oral health needs of the elderly? It is of vital import that we are well-trained and competent in executing a wide range of dental interventions as well as being especially understanding, compassionate, and aware of the special needs of the aging population. Within our profession, clinical knowledge is progressing at an exciting pace with the promise that we are continuously developing improved materials, better techniques, and refined capabilities to better preserve or improve oral function. Are we as current and skilled as we need to be? Are we ready for this "senior tsunami?"

Professor Alex Mersel, an internationally respected authority in geriatric dentistry, is the editor and author of several chapters within this significant new book titled *Treatment Dilemmas for Vulnerable Patients in Oral Health*. This resource is directed towards teaching dentists how they can better provide evidence-based dental treatment for their aging patients. Prof. Mersel has also assembled an outstanding cadre of chapter authors who represent true gerodontic expertise in their respective disciplines. Together they examine such salient concerns as oral/systemic relationships, periodontology, endodontics, neurologic/psychologic dimensions, masticatory function and nutrition, diagnosis and treatment of destructive caries, minimally invasive restorative dentistry approaches, removable and fixed prosthodontics considerations, and prevention strategies.

Geriatric dentistry requires from the practitioner the best of clinical, psychological, and social skills and demands an integrated and collaborative approach. With these chapters providing expert guidance, dental professionals will have the opportunity to significantly expand their clinical capabilities for oral rehabilitation.

This text also effectively utilizes a case-based approach recognizing that we often learn how to best care for our patients from our involvement with and observation of real cases. By considering authentic, complex, and multifaceted patient circumstances, a valuable "real-life" framing is created that promotes deeper engagement and authentic learning.

University of Colorado at Health Sciences Center   Douglas Berkey
Aurora, CO, USA

Foreword

Professor Alex Mersel in an authority in the field of geriatric dentistry. He is the editor and author of several chapters in the book entitled *Treatment Dilemmas for Vulnerable Patients in Oral Health*. He is specialized in prosthodontics at the Hadassah Faculty of Dental Medicine. He is also the founder and Chairman of the European College of Gerodontology (1994), Chairman of the FDI Section of Gerodontology (1997–1999), and Director of the FDI for the Europe Continuing Education Program (2013–2018).

Professor Alex Mersel has served as Director of the Geriatric Dentistry Studies, Department of Community Dentistry, at the Hadassah Faculty of Dental Medicine. He has published many scientific articles and chapters in various textbooks.

Grouping together authors presenting a true gerodontic expertise in their respective specialties, the authors invited to participate have reported on different chapters including the following topics: demography and aging, systemic diseases and oral health of elderly patients, physiological changes in endodontic, temporomandibular joint disorders in the elderly, masticatory function and nutritional status, carious destruction of the remaining teeth: diagnostic and treatment, minimal approaches for conservative restorations, evaluation of transitional or immediate complete dentures, limits of complete denture rehabilitation, and implant-supported overdenture: benefits and risks. In addition to the chapters already published, elderly patients are facing many problems. The first book constitutes a very complete panorama of geriatric dentistry, requiring multifaceted and collaborative approaches. The second book should include a review of endocrine and exocrine disorders, the conventional treatment, aiming to deliver a perfect treatment, reaching excellency and gold standard. This is in continuity and adds with creative innovation, aiming to treat both handicapped but also neglected patients.

Paris, France   Michel Goldberg

Contents

About the Authors

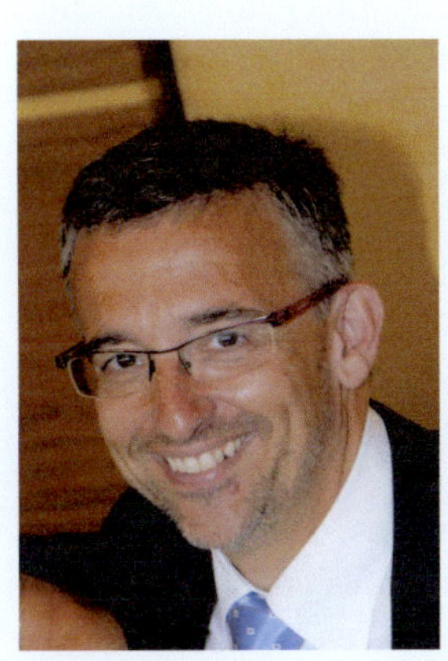

Subira Carles, MD, DDS, PhD

- Diplomate in Clinical Periodontology. Göteborg University.
- Associate professor, Faculty of Dentistry, Universitat de Barcelona.
- Director of the MS Degree of Adult Comprehensive Dentistry. University of Barcelona.
- Investigator of the IDI-BELL Institute, School of Dentistry, University of Barcelona, Barcelona, Spain.
- Implant Surgeon at the Dental Unit of Mataró's Public Hospital in Barcelona.

Dental & Oral Department, Faculty of Medicine and Health Sciences, School of Dentistry, Universitat de Barcelona, Barcelona, Spain

Gil Zvi Eisenberg, DMD

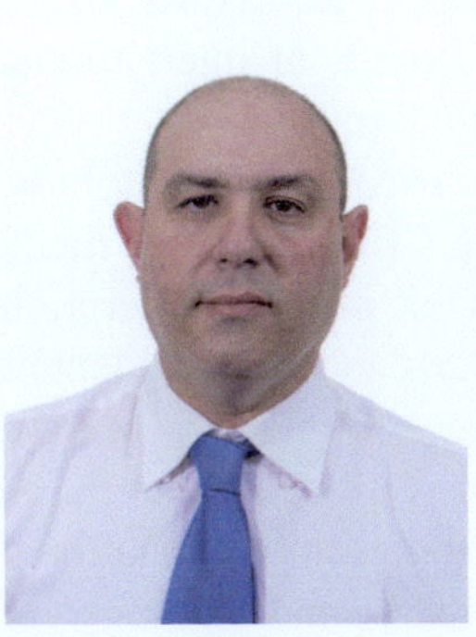

- Borne in Jerusalem 9/4/63.
- Married + 2.
- Home address: 4 Tapuach st. Motzza Illite.
- Clinic address: 96A Hertzel Blvd Jerusalem. Main focus oral rehab.
- Graduate D.M.D. 1992 Hebrew University Dental School Hadassah Ein Karem.
- Graduate of a 4-year root for Gerodontics Joined venture of Oral Public Dental Health Dpt. Dental School Hadassah' Ein Karem and Yard Sarah foundation.
- Head doctor of Karen-Maccabi Dental Clinic in Ness Ziona, 1998–2004.
- Certified for General Anestesia dentistry and practices General Anesthesia dentistry in Maccabi-dent special dental clinic in Ramat Ha Hayal, Tel Aviv

Assuta Hospital, Tel-Aviv, Israel

Jerusalem, Israel

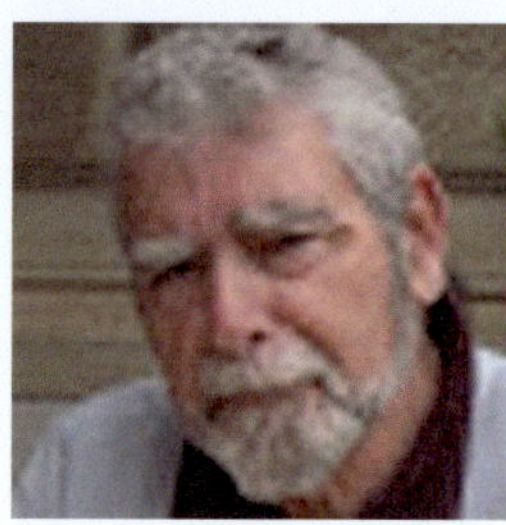

Michel Goldberg Born: 5 May 1938. He graduated in Paris and became dental surgeon in 1961, title obtained in the Medical Faculty of Paris. Doctor in Dental Sciences in 1973 (Université Paris V). Docteur d'Etat ès Sciences Naturelles (University Pierre et Marie Curie Paris VI. 1983). Associate Professor University Paris V (Université René Descartes—Paris V). Professor second class in Operative Dentistry. professor de 1ère class (October 1985) Professor de Categories Exceptionally in Biological Sciences—in May 1978.

He became Professor Emeritus with a first nomination in September 1, 2007, and furthermore, he was nominated in March 2010 (change from the dental school towards the medical faculty). In September 2011 he was nominated at the Medical Faculty (Sciences Biologiques et Biomédicales) (Paris 5—Université René Descartes). The third nomination was given in September 2015, and on September 4, 2019, he was nominated Emeritus for the 4 coming years.

International publications: He has published 244 articles (including editorials and articles), **two doctoral thesis** (Doctorate en sciences odontologiques and Doctorat d'Etat ès sciences naturelles). He has also published about 100 pedagogic articles in French. **Editor or co-editor** of 13 books and eight invited chapters in books. He is also a member of many editorial boards of international journals (dental and non-dental journals).

Chairman of the interface INSERM/Odontology. Member of the board of the CED-IADR for many years, he was the organizer of the Federation Dentaire Internationale in Paris and the president of the international conference in Nice of the International Association for Dental Research. He was the organizer of the 6th International Conference on the Chemistry and Biology of Mineralized Tissues. Last but not least, he has been President of the French Dental Association annual meeting.

Research interests: oral biology, tooth morphogenesis, amelogenesis, dentinogenesis, pulp biology, pulp regeneration, stem cells

Faculté des Sciences Fondamentales et Biomédicales, Paris, France
INSERM/Odontology, Paris, France
French Dental Association, Paris, France

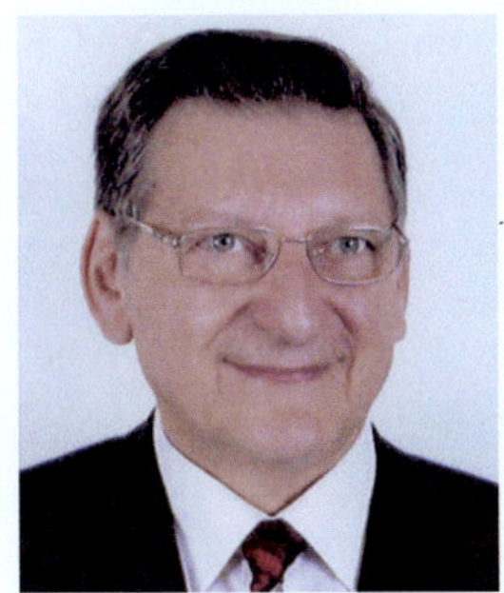

Alexander Mersel Alexandre Mersel (DOB: February 21, 1936) is an educationist, researcher, and specialist in prosthodontics. He received his graduation from the Faculty of Odontology, University of Lyon, France, in 1961 and specialized in prosthodontics, at the Hadassah Faculty of Dental Medicine, Hebrew University of Jerusalem, Israel, in 1979. With respect to his career, he has been Associate Professor at the Hadassah Faculty of Dental Medicine since 1992 and also Director of Complete Dentures Prosthodontics and Gerodontics studies (1978–1998) and Head of the Department of Removable Prosthodontics and Gerodontics at the Haifa Institute for Dental Advanced Studies (1986–1987). He also acted as consultant to the Prime Minister's commission of Public Health (1982) and Director of Dental Health Services Municipality of Jerusalem (1986–1988). He was also founder and Chairman of the European College of Gerodontology (1994), Convener and Chairman of FDI Section of Gerodontology (1997–1999), and Director of FDI for the Europe Continuing Education Program (2013–2018). He was a research fellow at Myers-JDC-Brookdale Institute of Jerusalem (1981) and was awarded The City of Paris Silver Medal (1986).

Currently, he serves as Director of the Geriatric Dentistry Studies, Department of Community Dentistry, at the Hadassah Faculty of Dental Medicine. He also serves as a member of the editorial board of several international journals. He is a member of the Academy of Dentistry International (ADI) and the Pierre Fauchard Academy (PFA). He published 102 scientific articles, three chapters in various textbooks, and recently, the book *Oral Rehabilitation for Compromised and Elderly Patients* (Springer, 2019).

Research interests: prosthodontics, gerodontics, complete dentures

Community Dentistry Hadassah School of Dental Medicine, University of Jerusalem, Jerusalem, Israel

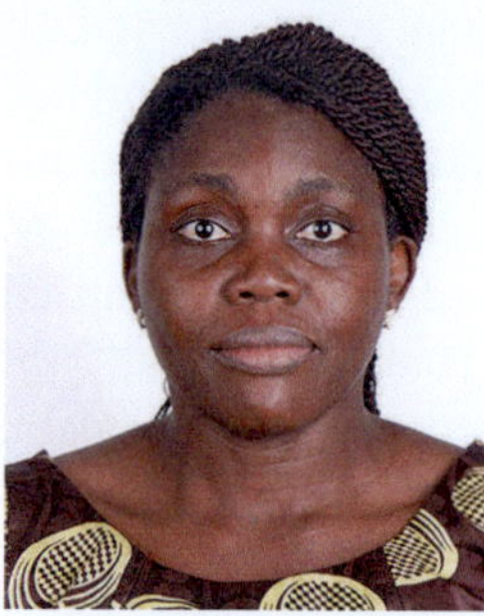

Akinboboye Bolanle Oyeyemi, BDS, FWACS, FCOI, MSc

Telephone:
- Home: +2348060599004
- Mobile: +2347057251024. +2348124197058

Post Held in the University:
Lecturer 1: 2012–2015:
- 400 L Departmental Course adviser
- Basic Clinical Skill departmental course coordinator
- Basic Dental Nursing Lecturer
- Member Curriculum committee
- Secretary exchange program committee, Faculty of Dental Sciences, College of Medicine, University of Lagos

Senior Lecturer: 2015–2018:
- 400 L Departmental Course adviser
- Basic Dental Nursing Lecturer
- Faculty 600L Course Adviser
- Faculty Examination Officer
- Member of University of Lagos Central Examination Committee
- University of Lagos Research Adjunct
- Faculty representative Academic Staff Union Committee

2018 to Date
- Being Assessed for Associate Professor

Post Held Outside University:
- Treasurer, International Association for Dental Research (IADR) Nigerian subdivision
- Financial Secretary, Nigerian Association of Restorative Dentist (NISORD) 2018 to date
- Protocol Officer in Medical Women Association, Lagos, 2011 till 2014
- Treasurer in Nigeria Medical Association (Lagos Chapter), August 2012 to 2014
- Assistant treasurer, West African Chapter of FCOI, August 2011–2013
- Vice Chairperson, Ogun State Medical Student Association, University of Ibadan, 1997–1998
- Member of Editorial Board, Ogun State Medical Student Association, University of Ibadan, 1996–1997
- Assistant Senior Prefect, Our Lady of Apostles Secondary School, Ogun, 1991

Membership:
- Member, International Association for Dental Research
- Member, Nigerian Dental Association

- Fellow, West African College of Surgeons
- Associate Fellow, National Postgraduate Medical College of Nigeria
- Fellow of College of Oral Implantologist
- Member of the Implant Prosthetic Section of the ICOI
- Member, Medical Women Association of Nigeria
- Member Nigeria Medical Association
- Member, NISORD

Services:

- Teaching undergraduate student
- Teaching of dental students on clinical postings
- Reviewer for many dental journals
- Moderation of weekly seminars for interns and residents
- Community outreach especially the elderly

Education:

- Senior Secondary School Leaving Certificate 1991
- Our Lady of Apostles Sec. School, Ijebu Ode, Ogun State, Nigeria (from 1985 to 1991)
- Bachelor of Dental Surgery [B.D.S.] 1999
- University of Ibadan, Ibadan, Oyo State, Nigeria (from 1991 to 1999)
- Fellow of West African College of Surgeons (from 2005 to May 2011)
- Lagos University Teaching Hospital
- Fellow College of Oral Implantologist
- M.Sc. Public Health (Health Management)
- University of Lagos 2016–2017

Work Experience:

- Housemanship, Lagos University Teaching Hospital (June 1999–June 2000)
- NYSC, Adeoyo State Hospital, Maxillofacial Unit, Ring Road, Ibadan, Oyo (2000–2001)
- Dental Officer, Nabille Dental Surgery, Dolphin, Lagos (Nov 2001–Feb 2003)
- Dental Officer, Hygeia Dental & Eye Clinic, Lagos (Feb 2003–Jul 2004)
- Dental Officer, St. Emmanuel Hospital, Isolo, Lagos (Oct 2004–June 2005)
- Residency program in Lagos University Teaching Hospital, Idi Araba
- Lecturer, University of Lagos
- External examiner, University of Maiduguri (2016–2018)

- External examiner, Obafemi Awolowo University (2019)
- External examiner, University of Nigeria (2019)
- External examiner, University of Calabar (2019)

Seminar/Community Work:

- Oyo NYSC & HCI "Iseyin Health Facility" Outreach. 2000
- Seminar titled "SMOKING CESSATION" organized by Oyo State Ministry of Health in collaboration with Lola Marhino Non-Governmental Organization. 2001
- Community outreach for the older population organized by the Department of Community Health, Faculty of Clinical Sciences, University of Lagos.

Research Grants/Award:

- University of Lagos Central research committee grant award for research titled "Is denture plaque a risk for aspiration pneumonia in the elderly?" (2019).

Publications:

- Ehizele A, Azodo C, Umoh A, Akinboboye B. Attitude of dental students to tobacco cessation services. Int J Dent Sci. 2009;7(1):1.
- Azodo C, Akinboboye B. Removable partial denture use amongst a selected group of Nigerian undergraduates. Eur J Gen Dent. 2012;1(1):30–3.
- Azodo CC, Odai CD, Akinboboye B, Azodo PA. Infection control in dental laboratories: a survey of Nigerian Dental Technology Students. Ebonyi Med J. 2012;11:37–42.
- Ajayi O, Akinboboye B. The choice of impression material among dentist. Niger Dent J. 2012;20:27–30.
- Akinboboye BO, Akeredou PA, Ogunrinde O, Sofola O, Oremosu O. Utilization of teeth replacement service among the elderly attending teaching hospitals in Lagos, Nigeria. Ann Health Med Sci. 2014;3:3.
- Akinboboye B, Shaba O, Akeredolu P, Oderinu O. Sociodemographic determinants of usage of complete denture in a Nigerian teaching hospital; a pilot study. Eur J Prosthodont. 2013;1:37–41.

- Akinboboye B, Azodo C, Soroye M. Partial edentulism and prosthetic unmet needs in a group of Nigerian Undergraduates. Odontostomatol Trop. 2014;37:48–52.
- Akeredolu P, Akinboboye B, Gbotolorun O, Emeka C, Adesida A. Management of dental anxiety: a survey of Nigerian dentists. Sahel Med J. 2014;17:47–52.
- Akinboboye BO, Ajayi YO, Umesi DC. Transcultural perception of maxillary midline diastema. Int J Esthet Dent. 2015;10:594–602.
- Akinboboye BO, Emeka CC, Shaba OP, Akeredolu PA, Olojede OI, Jokomba. Prosthetic rehabilitation of maxillofacial defect: The Lagos University Teaching Hospital Experience. Niger Q J Hosp Med. 2014;25:32–7.
- Akinboboye BO, Oderinu OH, Akeredolu PA, Shaba OP. Factors contributing to dissatisfaction of complete dentures. Niger Q J Hosp Med. 2014;25:38–42.
- Akinboboye B, Akeredolu PA, Akinsola OJ. Salivary viscosity and satisfaction in complete denture therapy. Niger Q Hosp Med J. 2015;25(1):1–4.
- Akinboboye BO, Ehizele AO, Temitope E. Influence of sociodemographic factors on perception of midline diastema. Niger Dent J. 2015;23:122–9.
- Akeredolu PA, Akinsola OJ, Akinboboye BO, Ekwenibe U. Knowledge and utilization patterns of information technology among healthcare personnel in Lagos University Teaching Hospital, Lagos. Niger Dent J. 2015;23:135–42.
- Ajayi YO, Akinboboye BO, Dosumu OO, Akeredolu PA. Awareness of dental implants among dental patients in Nigeria. J Med Biomed Res. 2016;15:40–8.
- Akinboboye BO, Sulaiman AO, Bamigboye SA, Akeredolu AA, Dosumu OO. Preliminary survey of impact of tooth loss on individuals with unrestored partially edentulous arch in southwestern Nigeria. Afr J Biomed Res. 2016;19:149–53.
- Ajayi YO, Akinboboye BO. Reasons for failure and replacement of Class I and Class II amal-

gam restorations in permanent teeth. Ann Biomed Sci. 2016;2:74–9.

- Akinboboye BO, Ajayi YO, Azodo CC, Oluwaniyi SO. Prosthetic status and need of psychiatric patients. Niger J Restorat Dent. 2016;1:48–51.
- Akinboboye BO, Mersel A, Akeredolu PA. Relating formal, informal religious activities with complete denture satisfaction. Niger J Dent Res. 2017;2(1):37–42.
- Akinboboye BO, Akeredolu PA, Oderinu OH. Relationship between satisfaction with complete denture and basal seat characteristics: A pilot study. Niger J Restorat Dent. 2017;2:6–9.
- Akinboboye BO, James O, Azodo CC, Adekunle AA, Oluwaniyi SO. Oral health status and treatment needs in – patients of a Nigerian Psychiatric Hospital. Niger J Dent Res. 2018;3:28–32.
- Akinboboye BO, Ajayi YO, Azodo CC. Oral health status and diet habit of institutionalised elder group. Ann Biomed Sci. 2018;3:44–54. www.ajol.info/index.php/abs/article/view/168976.
- Esan TA, Akinboboye BO, Olusile AO. Social characteristics and motivation of patients attending a removable prosthodontics clinic in Ile – Ife, Nigeria. Niger J Restorat Dent. 2017;2:36–41.
- Akinboboye BO, Ogunyemi AO, Ladi-Akinyemi TW. Oral health status and service utilization among a group of rural older Nigerians. Afr J Oral Health. 2017;7:24–31.
- Ajayi YO, Akinboboye BO. Evaluation of aesthetic outcome of single tooth implant borne restoration. Niger J Dent Res. 2018:31–6.
- Ajayi YO, Nwachukwu N, Akinboboye BO. Treatment outcome of short dental implants. J W Afr Coll Surg. 2017;7:52–71.
- Akinboboye BO. Treatment needs, association of missing and replaced tooth among older population in a rural setting. Niger J Dent Res. 2018;3:88–96.

- Akinboboye BO, Mersel A, Malomo B, Olawuyi A. Religiosity & self efficacy in complete denture wearer. Niger J Med Dent Educ. 2019;1:14–20.
- Akinboboye BO, Ogunkola AO, Ayedun OS, Akeredolu PA, Oredugba FA. Presentation and management of ectodermal dysplasia: A case report. ULJDS. 2018;2:41–6.
- Adenuga-Taiwo OA, Akinboboye BO, Awotile AO. Prosthetic experience of teaching and learning of fabrication of removable partial denture among the Nigerian Dental schools. University of Lagos. J Dent Sci. 2019;3(1):1.

Dissertation:

- Demand and uses of complete denture: a year follow up (Dissertation for the award of fellow of West African College of Surgeons).
- Self and Professional Oral Health Care Among the Elderly in Ado-Odo/Ota LGA, Ogun State. Dissertation for the award of M.Sc. Public Health (Health Management).

Conference Presentations:

- Ehizele AO, Azodo CC, Umoh A, **Akinboboye B**. Compliance with as approach in tobacco cessation services among Nigerian dental students. In program and abstract of the 6th Annual General Meeting and Scientific Conference of Nigeria Medical Association Edo state branch, Benin City, Nigeria, July 14–16, 2010.
- Ehizele AO, Azodo CC, Umoh A, **Akinboboye B**. Attitude of dental students to tobacco cessation services. Abstract number 2480. In program and abstract of the 87th General Session & Exhibition of the IADR, Miami Beach Convention Center in Miami, Florida, April 1–4, 2009.
- **Akinboboye B**, Akeredolu P, Sofola O, Oremosu O, Ogunrinde TJ. Profile of Geriatric Patient attending Prosthetic Out Patient Clinic. In program and abstract of 4th Scientific Conference of School of Dental Sciences College of Medicine University of Lagos.
- Ogunkola A, **Akinboboye B**, Oredugba O, Akeredolu P. A case report of ectodermal dysplasia. In program and abstract of 4th Scientific Conference of School of Dental Sciences College of Medicine University of Lagos.

- **Akinboboye B**, Shaba OP, Akeredolu PA, Oderimu OH. Demand and use of complete denture. In program and abstract of IADR/AMER, Abuja September 2011.
- **Akinboboye B, Azodo C, Soroye M.** Partial edentulism and unmet prosthetics needs amongst young adult Nigerian. In program and abstract of 2nd Annual Scientific Conference of the School of Dentistry College of Medical Sciences, University of Benin.
- **Akinboboye B**, Shaba OP., Akeredolu PA, Oderimu OH. Relationship between satisfaction with complete dentures and basal seat characteristics. FDI 2013 conference, Istanbul Turkey.
- **Akinboboye B,** Ehizele A, Esan T. Influence of sociodemographics factors on perception of midline diastema. IADR conference, Cape Town, June 2014.
- **Akinboboye B,** Ogunyemi AO. Prevalence of oral diseases and access to oral health care amongst elderly in rural area. First National Conference on Inclusivity, Equality and Diversity in University Education in Nigeria, September, 2017.
- **Akinboboye B,** Ogunyemi AO. Cleaning aids—twigs, diet and low caries prevalence in the seniors. IADR Conference. London 2018.
- **Akinboboye B,** Ogunyemi AO. Need and demand of dental care in an older population.

Courses Attended:

- Mini residency styled dental implant course by Caribbean Institute of Oral and Maxillofacial Implantology and Surgery.
- Manuscripts writing workshop organized by West African College of physicians.
- Commonwealth Dental Association regional workshop on restorative materials in a resource-limited setting.
- Research methodology in medicine workshop organized by National Postgraduate Medical College of Nigeria.
- Atraumatic restoration workshop.
- Dental implants with hands-on training organized by Dental Solutions.
- Responsible conduct of research and grant writing organized by MEDU, September 2013.

- CMUL/MEPIN Bioethics Workshop by Research management Office. Alumni Hall. February 11, 2015.
- Training of course advisers and examination officer organized by the University of Lagos.
- Short Implant course organized by Clinical Support Services Limited, April 2015.
- Oral B CME/CDP workshop organized by Cardinal Academy in Partnership with Oral B, May 2015.
- Female Health Care Access to Finance Entrepreneurship Breakfast Meeting organized by Access Bank Plc. April 30, 2015.
- NHREC Guidelines/Electronic Protocol Review Training organized by Building Research and Innovation in Nigeria's Science (BRAINS). October 10, 2016.
- Workshop on Public Health Research in Infectious Diseases, May 8–12, 2017.
- National Conference on Inclusivity, Equality and Diversity in University Education in Nigeria, 12–13 September 2017.

Personal Data:
- Date of Birth: 30 May 1974
- Place of Birth: Sagamu, Ogun State, Nigeria
- Marital Status: Married with three children with ages 13, 10, and 9 years.

Hobbies:
- Reading, Music, and Traveling

Referees:
Prof. G. T. Arotiba:
- Dean of Faculty Dental Sciences,
- College of Medicine,
- University of Lagos, Lagos.

Prof. T. Esan:
- Department of Restorative Dentistry
- Faculty of Dental Sciences,
- College of Health Sciences,
- Obafemi Awolowo University.

Prof. O. O. Dosumu:
- Department of Restorative Dentistry,
- Faculty of Dental Sciences,
- College of Medicine,
- University of Ibadan,
- Oyo State

Department of Restorative Dentistry, Faculty of Dental Sciences, College of Medicine, University of Lagos, Lagos, Nigeria

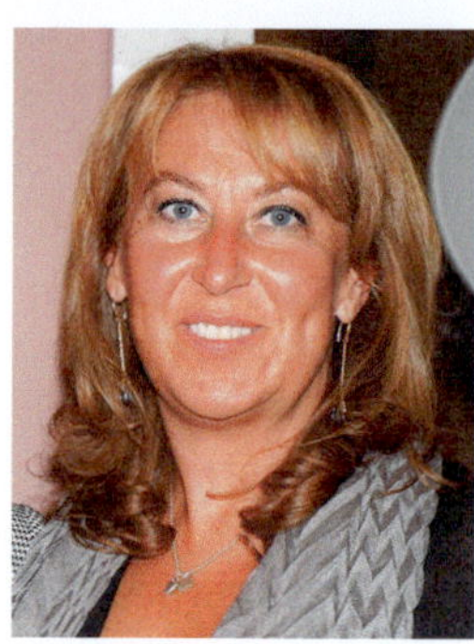

Marzia Segù, DDS, MS, PhD

- **Specialist in Orthodontics.**
  - PhD in Experimental Surgery and Microsurgery.
  - Education Program Director of the Degree in Dental Hygiene at the University of Pavia.
  - Currently, she holds teaching in Temporomandibular Disorders, at the School of Dentistry, University of Pavia.
  - In January 2014, the Italian Ministry of University and Research (MIUR) appointed her as an Associate Professor by scientific merit.
  - Instructor of the "Advanced Course in Edgewise Mechanics" at the Charles H. Tweed Foundation Tucson (AZ), USA.
  - Regular Member of the Charles H. Tweed International Foundation for Orthodontic Research.
  - Referee of the "Cochrane Oral Health Group" Manchester for Temporomandibular Disorders."
  - Full member and Past National Representative for Italy in the Council of the European Academy of Craniomandibular Disorders (EACD).
  - Past President of the Italian Society of Dentistry in Sleep Medicine (SIMSO) and of the Italian Society for Oro Facial Pain and TMD (SIDA).
  - Member of the European Continuing Education Program for East Europe for temporomandibular disorders, orofacial pain, and dentistry in sleep medicine.
  - President of the local section of the Italian Society of Dentistry (AIO).
  - Italian Board of Orthodontics (IBO) Certificate.
  - Ordinary member of the Italian Society of Orthodontics (SIDO)

  Universita di Milano, Milano, Italy

Universita di Pavia, Pavia, Italy

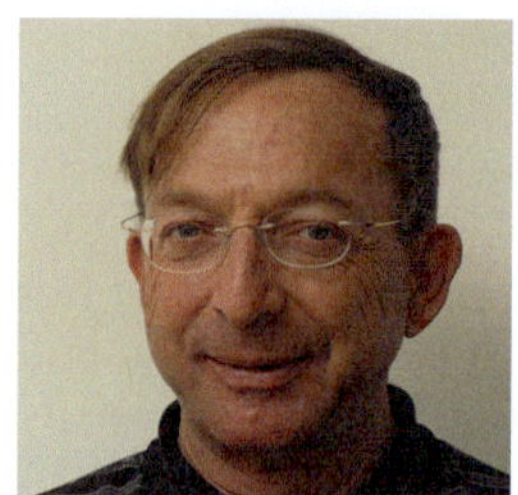

Joseph Shapira

1. Personal Details:

- Date of birth: August 15, 1946
- Country of Birth: Israel
- Identity number: 3911104
- Nationality: Israeli
- Family status: Married + 3

- Military service: Armored forces
- Permanent address: My home address is:
15 Vormiza St. Appt. # 73, Tel Aviv, Israel 6264214
- Tel # 972508670162
- Email: shapiraj@cc.huji.ac.il, josephsha@ekmd.huji.ac.il

2. Higher Education:

- 1967–1973: The Hebrew University—Hadassah Faculty of Dental Medicine, Jerusalem, Israel. Graduated with distinction. DMD Thesis with Prof. Heling B. #5.
- 1974: D.M.D. degree.
- 1977–1979: Postgraduate and residency program specializing in Dentistry for Children, with special emphasis on Dentistry for the Handicapped and High-Risk Patients, The Children's Hospital of Philadelphia, University of Pennsylvania. Preceptors were: M. M. Album, R. Johnson, and J. L. Ackerman. Research project: "Detection of a fibroblast proliferation inhibitory factor from *Capnocytophaga sputigena*" in collaboration with Drs. J. Rosenblum, R. H. Stevens, and M. Sela (Published: Inf. & Immun, 1980 #8).
- 1979: Board Eligible in Pediatric Dentistry—The American Academy of Pediatric Dentistry.
- 1979: Specialist in Pediatric Dentistry (Ministry of Health, Israel).

Non-academic Studies:

- 1966–1967: Economics and Political Sciences (1 year), The Hebrew University of Jerusalem.
- 1966: Course in Computers planning and programming (6 months).
- 1974–1977: In-Service Training—The Department of Pediatric Dentistry, The Hebrew University—Hadassah Faculty of Dental Medicine.
- 1975: General Anesthesia Course (3 months), Tel-Hashomer Hospital, Tel-Aviv.
- 1985: Summer workshop: "Oral care of the institutionalized patients" and "Dental treatment of disabled patients in intramural and extramural clinics"—University of Washington, Seattle: The Dental Education for Care of the Disabled Program.

3. Appointments at the Hebrew University:

- 1974: Instructor (full time) in the Department of Pediatric Dentistry, The Hebrew University—Hadassah Faculty of Dental Medicine.
- 1979: Lecturer and staff member in the Department of Pediatric Dentistry, The Hebrew University—Hadassah Faculty of Dental Medicine.
- 1984: Senior clinical lecturer in Pediatric Dentistry, The Hebrew University—Hadassah Faculty of Dental Medicine.
- 1985: Senior lecturer in Pediatric Dentistry, The Hebrew University—Hadassah Faculty of Dental Medicine.
- 1993: Associate Clinical Professor in Pediatric Dentistry, The Hebrew University—Hadassah Faculty of Dental Medicine.
- 1996: Associate Professor in Pediatric Dentistry, The Hebrew University—Hadassah Faculty of Dental Medicine.
- 2008: Professor in Pediatric Dentistry, The Hebrew University—Hadassah Faculty of Dental Medicine.

4. Additional Functions/Tasks at the Hebrew University:

- 1980: Established the Unit of Dental Treatment for Handicapped and Special Care Patients, Department of Pediatric Dentistry, Hebrew University—Hadassah School of Dental Medicine.
- 1980: Consultant in Pediatric Dentistry, Cleft-Palate team, The Hebrew University—Hadassah Medical Center, Jerusalem.
- 1988–1993: Editor-in-Chief, The Official Quarterly Journal of the Faculty of Dental Medicine in Jerusalem and Alumni (for 5 years).
- 1998–2002: Director, The Unit for Dental Treatment of Developmental Disabilities and High-Risk Pediatric Patients, Department of Pediatric Dentistry, The Hebrew University—Hadassah School of Dental Medicine.
- 2000–2002: Director, Post-Graduate Studies in Pediatric Dentistry, Department of Pediatric Dentistry, Hebrew University—Hadassah School of Dental Medicine.
- 2001–2003: Member of the Senate of the Hebrew University.

- 2002–2014: Chairman of the Department of Pediatric Dentistry, The Hebrew University—Hadassah School of Dental Medicine.
- 2014: Volunteer in the Department of Pediatric Dentistry, The Hebrew University—Hadassah School of Dental Medicine.

Membership in Faculty Committees:

- 1987–1988: Member, Scientific Committee—The World Dental Congress Jerusalem.
- 1990–1993: Member of the Teachers—Students Committee, Hebrew University—Hadassah Faculty of Dental Medicine.
- 1990–1993: Tutor of the sixth year dental students.
- 1990–1993: Member of the Committee for Evaluation of Para-Medical Studies, Hebrew University—Hadassah Faculty of Dental Medicine.
- 1991–2001: Member of the Admission Committee, Hebrew University—Hadassah Faculty of Dental Medicine.
- 1994–1997: Member of the Pedagogic Committee, Hebrew university—Hadassah Faculty of Dental Medicine.
- 1994–1997: Member of the Sub-committee of the Admission Committee for the Acceptance of candidates for advanced years, Hebrew University—Hadassah Faculty of Dental Medicine.
- 1994–1997: Member of the Committee for Continuing Education Courses, Hebrew University—Hadassah Faculty of Dental Medicine.
- 1996–1999: Member of the Committee for Academic Development, Hebrew University—Hadassah Faculty of Dental Medicine.
- 1999–2002: Member the Committee for Clinical Equipment and Infrastructure, Hebrew University—Hadassah Faculty of Dental Medicine.
- 1999–2001: Chairman, The Committee for the Development and Improvement of Clinical Services, Hebrew University—Hadassah Faculty of Dental Medicine.
- 2002–2005: Member of the Teaching Committee, Hebrew University—Hadassah Faculty of Dental Medicine.

- 2005–2013: Member of the Admission Committee, Hebrew University—Hadassah Faculty of Dental Medicine.
- 2005–2013: Chairman, the Pedagogic Committee, Hebrew University—Hadassah Faculty of Dental Medicine.
- 2007–2013: Chairman, the Committee for promotion to Lecture track, Hebrew University—Hadassah Faculty of Dental Medicine.

5. Service in Other Academic and Research Institutions:

- 1988: Visiting Professor of Pediatric Dentistry—**University of Pennsylvania**, The Children's Hospital of Philadelphia (3 months).
- 1992: Visiting Professor in Pediatric Dentistry—**Harvard School of Dental Medicine**, Children's Hospital, Boston (2.5 months).
- 1998: Visiting Professor in Pediatric Dentistry—**The University of Sydney**, Westmead Hospital & Dental School, Australia (6 weeks—lectures, seminars, and clinical activities).
- 1998: Visiting Professor in Pediatric Dentistry—**The Nippon Dental University** in Niigata and Tokyo, Japan (4 weeks—lectures, seminars, and clinical activities).
- 2008: Visiting Professor in Pediatric Dentistry—**The University of Sao-Paulo** in Brazil (4 weeks—lectures, seminars, and clinical activities).
- 2012: Visiting Professor in Pediatric Dentistry—**The University of New York** (4 weeks—lectures, seminars, and clinical activities).
- 2014: Visiting Professor in Pediatric Dentistry—**The University of New York** (4 weeks—lectures and clinical activities).

6. Other Activities:

- 1988–1991: Advisor to the "Jerusalem Variety Center for Child and Family Development"—The Dental Project.
- 1988–1993: Consultant to the DVI—("Dental Volunteers for Israel")—A dental clinic, free of charge, for underprivileged children of Jerusalem.

- 1989–Today: Senior Dental Consultant to "Elwin," the largest Institution for People with Mental Retardation in the Jerusalem area.
- 1988: Advisor to "Akim"—Association for the Habilitation of People with Mental Disabilities in Israel. Ad-hoc committee: Meeting the dental needs and demands of people with mental retardation in Israel.
- 1992: Organizing committee: The Israel Society for Sedation, Analgesia and Dental Anesthesia.
- 1992: Member of a Joint Committee: The Dental Schools in Israel & The Ministry of Health on "Guidelines for the use of Sedation in Dentistry."
- 1993–1994: Acting head, The Unit of Dental Treatment for Patients with Handicap and Special Needs Care.
- 1993–1998: Member of the Examining Committee for Specializing in Orthodontics— The Scientific Council of the Israel Dental Association.
- 1994–2000: Member of the Examining Committee for Specializing in Pediatric Dentistry—The Scientific Council of the Israel Dental Association.
- 1993: Scientific Committee of the annual meeting of the Israel Dental Association.
- 1995–1996: Appointed by the Ministry of Labour and Welfare to conduct: A National Survey: The Oral Health Status and Dental Needs of the Population with Mental Retardation in Israel.
- 1996–2006: Member of the Professional Committee for Specializing in Pediatric Dentistry—The Scientific Council of the Israel Dental Association.
- 1998–Today: Appointed as an Advisor of the Editorial Board of *Asian Journal of Cancer*.
- 1999–Today: Member of the Editorial Board of "Adkan"—Israel Dental Update. Member of the organizing committee, 9th International Dental Congress on Modern Pain Control.
- 1998: Appointed by the Ministry of Health— member of a committee for "The proper and reasonable use of fluoridated dentifrice."
- 2001: Invited to conduct a 2 day course by the National Center for Orofacial Disorders,

Gothenburg, Sweden, on "Comprehensive Multidisciplinary Team Approach: Pedodontic–Orthodontic for the Dental Treatment of Special Needs Children" (Sept. 2001).

- 2005: Appointed by the Scientific Council of the Israeli Dental Association—member of a committee for the evaluation of The Guidelines written by the Ministry of Health on "The Use of Sedation and General Anesthesia in the Dental Clinic."
- 2006: Appointed by the Ministry of Health— member of a committee for the implementation of the recommendations made by the investigators of the death of a 2-year-old boy in a dental clinic.
- 2013: Appointed as member of the "International Sedation Task Force" by the International Association of Pediatric Dentistry (IAPD).
- 2015: Appointed as the Head of SHALVA's Oral Hygiene Training program (OHTC). Shalva is an Association for Mentally and Physically Challenged Children that provides a unique composite of all-encompassing therapeutic, educational, and recreational care for 500 individuals with varying disabilities from infancy to young adulthood.
- 2018: Appointed as the A professional Director of the Project providing dental health services for students in Israel from the age of 5 (kindergarten) to the age of 15 (more than million pupils), on behalf and funded by the Ministry of Health, the Federation of local authorities in Israel, and by FemiPrimium, which specializes in providing health services in Israel. The project provides health services to students in Israel oral hygiene training, oral and dental health care, fluoride varnish applications for the kindergarten kids, and dmf/DMFT survey for age 5 and 12.

Prizes and Awards:

- 1973: Outstanding achievements and performance in undergraduate studies in pediatric dentistry. Award by the American Society of Dentistry for Children.
- 1973: Recipient of the M. Albert Award for excellent achievements as senior year under-

graduate student at the Hebrew University—Hadassah Faculty of Dental Medicine.

- 1976: Prize for best research article, the American Society of Dentistry for Children (Co-author). #1
- 1985: Prize for best research article, the American Society of Dentistry for Children (Co-author). #11
- 1994: Outstanding teacher, Faculty of Dental Medicine, The Hebrew University.
- 1995: Outstanding teacher, Faculty of Dental Medicine, The Hebrew University.
- 1998: Outstanding teacher, Rector's list for excellence in teaching, The Hebrew University.
- 1999: Outstanding teacher, Faculty of Dental Medicine, The Hebrew University.
- 2000: Outstanding teacher, Faculty of Dental Medicine, The Hebrew University.
- 2006: Outstanding teacher, Faculty of Dental Medicine, The Hebrew University.
- 2014: Outstanding teacher, Rector's list for excellence in teaching, The Hebrew University.

7. Research Grants:

- Clinical and microbiological effects of chlorhexidine and arginine sustained-release varnishes in the mentally retarded. Perio-Products Co. Ltd. 1993–1994 (**Shapira J***, Sela MN and Goultschin J)—$2500, **#37, 44.**
- National survey of the dental needs of Israel's population with mental retardation. Ministry of Labour and Welfare, 1995–1996 (**Shapira J*** and Mann J)—$21,400, **#55.**
- A grant given by "Keren Haezvonot (Apotropos)" for High Risk & Special Need Dental Patients, 2001 (**Shapira J**, Holan G, Kochavi D)—100,000 IS.
- The relationship between the salivary secretory immune system and periodontal disease in Down syndrome individuals. Dr. Izador I. Cabakoff Research Endowment Fund. 2002–2004 (Bachrach G*, Chaushu S* and **Shapira J**)—$10,000—Presented in the IADR Meeting, 2005. **# A-34.**
- A grant given by "ILAN—Israel Foundation for Handicapped Children" for the Study of the dental and oral status of cerebral palsied individuals, the prevalence of traumatized injuries teeth among them, and the delivery of a com-

prehensive multidisciplinary dental treatment for them—"Ilanot project," 2003–Today (**Shapira J*** and Peretz B (adjunct)—120,000 IS). **#65.**

- A grant given by "Ashalim"—The Association for Planning & Development of Services for Children and Youth at Risk & their Families, 2004–2005 (**Shapira J***)—37,500 IS.
- Assessing the caries risk of children undergoing orthodontic treatment. Ivoclar Vivadent AG, Lichtensrein, 2004–2005 (Katz-Sagi H*, **Shapira J*,** Steinberg D, Redlich M, Peretz B*)—Research Grant equivalent to 14,700 IS. Presented in the IADR meeting, 2005. **# A-35, A-39.**
- A grant given by "Hakeren Hameshutefet"— The Hebrew University and The Hadassah Medical Center: calcium-phosphor balance in children and adolescent patients suffering from renal failure, 2005–2006 (Davidovich E*, Smith P, Peretz B, Aframian DJ, **Shapira J**)— 10,000 IS.
- A grant given by Ministry of Health-Chief Scientist: Saliva as a possible predictive diagnostic tool for disturbances in calcium-phosphor balance in children and adolescent patients suffering from renal failure, 2005– 2006 (Davidovich E*, Smith P, Peretz B, Aframian DJ, **Shapira J**)—20,000 IS. # **A-37.**
- A grant given by The Ted Arison Family Foundation for (1) Comprehensive Dental Health Program for 80 Pediatric Cancer Patients. (2) Salivary Microorganisms and Oral Status in Children Undergoing Oncology Treatment. (3) Oral Health and Pain in Children Undergoing Cancer Chemotherapy: Impact on their Quality of Life. **Shapira J*,** Halperson E, Peretz B, Steinberg D, Gabarin N, Weintraub M—$70,908. Presented in the IADR meeting, 2006. # **A-38.**
- A research grant given by "GC Europe," 2007– 2008, for "An in vitro study of tooth mousse potential to induce remineralization of an initial enamel decay and to prevent demineralization of enamel in primary teeth"—(R. Bar-Hillel, M. Moskoviz, E. Mamber and **J. Shapira***), $7000.

- A Research grant in corporation with Alyn Hospital, 2008, for the study of "Calculus accumulation and the prevalence of caries in children fed via Gastrostom compared to that of children fed orally—Chemical and microbiological analysis of saliva." Moskovitz M, Cohen J, Hidas A, Beri M, Ben Dov E, Steinberg D, and **Shapira J**—$2000.
- A grant given by The Ted Arison Family Foundation 2008 for Comprehensive Dental Health Program for 80 Pediatric Cancer Patients. $47,000.
- A grant given by "Friends of Israel" in Canada, 2013, for Dental treatment of children with special needs treated in the Department of Pediatric Dentistry, Hebrew University—Hadassah School of Dental Medicine. **Shapira J and Stabholz A.** $500,000.

8. Teaching at the Hebrew University:

Supervision of Doctoral Degree Students:

Instructing DMD Theses:

- 1994–1995: Zadok Nili: The prevention of dental diseases among developmentally disabled patients—Audio-visual presentation. Co-supervisor—Prof. E. Bimstein.
- 1994–1995: Nabis Rivka: Morphologic parameters of the first premolar of children with Down syndrome in comparison to normal children. Co-supervisors—Prof. B. Peretz, Prof. P. Smith.
- 1995–1996: Katznel Vered: Morphologic parameters of the second deciduous molars in children with Down syndrome and in healthy children. Co-supervisors—Prof. B. Peretz, Prof. P. Smith. #50.
- 1999–2000: Petuchenko Andrei: Dental health status and dental needs of children with disabilities, studying in the special education system in the Jerusalem area.
- 2000–2001: Dvir Orit: A survey among parents of children with disabilities about their motivation, expectation and satisfaction with the results of the dental treatment rendered to their children.
- 2001–2002: Palmon-Katz Yael: Occlusal traits, sucking habits, the prevalence of otitis media and the relation between them among day-care children. Co-supervisors: Ben-Bassat Y.

- 2004–2006: Khury Samir: <u>Evaluation of propofol as a sedative agent in children during dental treatment.</u> Co-supervisor—Prof Peretz B.
- 2005–2006: Gabay Alona: <u>Validation of a questionnaire to measure children's and parental perceptions of child's oral health related quality of life</u>. Co-supervisors: Zusman S, Kushnir D, Ram D.
- 2006–2007: Knane Muhamad—Does chlorhexidine cleaning before fissure sealants application improve the conditions? (Dr. E. Davidovich, Dr. N. Beyth).
- 2007–2008: Ran Asher—Oral variables, sialochemistry and pH measurements among children with liver transplantation (Co—Dr. E. Davidovich and Dr. R. Shapira).
- 2007–2008: Mazor Sigal—Oral variables, sialochemistry and pH measurements among teenage girls with anorexia (Co—Dr. E. Davidovich and Dr. Y. Danzinger).
- 2007–2008: Nida Yonas—Early Childhood Caries: A survey among 1500 2–6 year old children of Ethiopian immigrants (Co—Prof. Peretz and Dr. E. Davidovich).
- 2007–2008: Ruth yaul-Agiv—A survey among 2–6 year old children of Ethiopian immigrants: anxiety, temperament and cooperative behavior during dental examination (Co—Prof. B. Peretz and Dr. E. Davidovich).
- 2007–2008: Neta Yanko—Dental trauma, oral habits and developmental defects among 1500 2–6 year old children of Ethiopian immigrants (Co—Dr. E. Davidovich).

<u>Reviewer of DMD Theses:</u>
- 1995: Giora Frenkel
- 1996: Amir Hadar
- 1998: Emanuel Achdut
- 2002: Ilan Hirsh
- 2003: Lilach Even-Paz
- 2003: Marwat Churi
- 2004: Masha Bongart
- 2005: Liat Shavit
- 2006: Machlev Shlomit
- 2006: Miri Bongart

<u>Instructing of the M.Sc. Theses:</u>
- 2002: Dr. Maora Zigmond, co-supervisors: Dr. S. Chaushu, Dr. G. Bachrach, Prof. E. Yefenof,

Prof. A. Becker, Prof. A. Stabholz. # Article submitted to Clinical Immunology, Feb 2005: "Age dependent deficiency in salivary antibodies secretion in Down syndrome."

Reviewer of M.Sc. Theses:
• 2002: Dr. Gali Peleg

Instructing for B.Sc. Theses:
• 2002: Bosiba Efrat
• 2002: Ben-Gal Gilad
• 2004: Gorin Yuliana
• 2004: Goldwine Uri
• 2004: Stark Tzachi
• 2004: Slobobinski Miri
• 2006: Tzach Rinat
• 2006: Dinoor Noam
• 2006: Mazor Sigal
• 2007: Rave-Ilan Lilach
• 2007: Udko Lisa
• 2007: Naama Hunny
• 2008: Orit Bliar

Instructing Basic Science Theses During Rotation in Postgraduate Specialty Studies in Pediatric Dentistry:
• 2000: Dr. Dan Lidar, Eating habits and food preference of children with pervasive developmental disorders.
• 2001: Dr. Giesela Bernstein, Teething as a medical problem—myth or reality? (#74).
• 2007: Dr. Rita Bar Hillel, An in vitro study of tooth mousse potential to induce remineralization of an initial enamel decay and to prevent demineralization of enamel in primary teeth.

Postdoctoral Fellows and Visitors:
• 2002–2004: Dr. Hanali Abu Shilbayih Abdlrahman—Fellow from Ramallah, The D. Walter Cohen Middle East Center for Continuing Education in Dentistry.
• 2005: Dr. Yasser Abu-Tair—Fellow from East Jerusalem, The D. Walter Cohen Middle East Center for Continuing Education in Dentistry.
• 2007: Dr. Hassan Nashasshibi—Fellow from Ramallah, The D. Walter Cohen Middle East Center for Continuing Education in Dentistry.

Courses Taught by Candidate:
Doctorate Courses (1996–Present):
• Lectures for the 5th senior year dental students on the subjects: Course # 97869

- Diagnosis and Treatment Planning for the Pediatric Dental Patient.
- Developmental Disturbances (color and shape) in the Formation of Teeth.
- Use of Sedation and General Anesthesia for the Pediatric Dental Patient.
- The Delivery of Dental Oral Care for Children with Disabilities.
- Clinical Teaching: Course # 97973
- Instructing students in the clinic during their last senior year of clinical studies in Pediatric Dentistry.

Dental Hygienists Course:
- Lectures for the senior year hygienist students on: Behavior management, oral health, and preventive measures for high-risk children with developmental disabilities.

Specialty Studies in Pediatric Dentistry:
- Courses in Sedation, Traumatology, Hospital Dentistry, and Dentistry for Special Need Patients.
- Clinical instruction during the delivery of emergencies, routine clinical work with sedatives and in the operating room under General Anesthesia.

Extracurricular Teaching (in the Last 5 Years):
- Preparation course for the Israeli National Board Examinations—Developmental Disturbances (Color and Shape) in the Formation of Teeth.
- Orthodontic Postgraduates Seminar: Conservative Approaches for the Treatment of Dental Caries. The Use of Fissure Sealants with or without Composite Resins.
- One-day course, Beit Izi Shapira for Developmentally Disabled Children, Raanana: "Preventive Oral Measures and Restorative Considerations of Dental Treatment for Developmentally Disabled Children."
- One-day course to the Dentists of The Ministry of Labour and Welfare on: "Behavior Management Techniques, including the Pharmacological Approach, in the Treatment of Patients with Mental Retardation."
- "Elwin" Institution for People with Mental Retardation.
- Department of Pediatrics, Mount Scopus, A seminar "Pediatric Dentistry for Pediatricians."

- One-day course to postgraduate dentists and dental hygienists on: "Comprehensive Multidisciplinary Team Approach for the Delivery of Dental Treatment to Children with Special Needs" and "Considerations in the Dental Treatment for Children with Developmental Disabilities."

Prof. Joseph Shapira was the Chairman of the Department of Pediatric Dentistry, Hebrew University—Hadassah Faculty of Dental Medicine, Jerusalem, Israel. Following his graduation with distinction in Jerusalem in 1974, he had specialized for 2 years in pediatric dentistry, with special emphasis on dentistry for special needs children, in The Children's Hospital of Philadelphia, University of Pennsylvania, USA.

Prof. Shapira is an expert in Dentistry for Special Needs and High-Risk Medically Compromised Patients as well as in the use of sedative agents regarding management of anxiety and behavior control

Department of Pediatric Dentistry, Hadassah University School of Dental Medicine, Jerusalem, Israel

Children's Hospital of Philadelphia, Philadelphia, PA, USA

Oral Health: Ethical and Clinical Concerns

Alexander Mersel and Subira Carles

1   Introduction

The demographic changes, the economic evolution, the technological revolution, and the education level are changing the profile of the patients. More and more individuals are looking for preventive and restorative solutions. Numerous barriers exist, increasing the number of neglected patients. In addition to the elderly cohorts, underserved children and handicapped persons also need special care. It is wishful to reduce this important gap. The consequences for our Profession are Ethical dilemmas between the "Best" and a "Poor" treatment. Our task as educators is to provide the practitioner with clinical approaches in order to be able to deliver the appropriate clinical solutions to their patients. Humanity was always curious to know; knowledge regarding science was the strongest trend in human beings! Faust was ready to sell his soul only for satisfying this passion. Loving a God or the devil only for progressing toward the absolute is the same sin of pride. Each society happens to possess a true and essential knowledge for our daily task which are to be accomplished. Kant classified three categories:

Ideological quality; infinity in the research of the best. Realistic quality; in relation to materiality; negative quality or wrong; bad interpretation.

He also noted the contradiction between quality and quantity. Of course, the trend to the Perfect and the Absolute provides a total conflictual situation. Therefore, Hegel introduced the approach of dialectics between the opposite sides; between one analysis and another must be some synthesis. The interference between two opposite imperative should conduct a new concept involving totally the two partners. In dentistry, the main partners are the patient and the dentist. The patient is expected to demonstrate a perfect cooperation with the dentist to supply the best treatment. To achieve this commitment, we have to underline that quality has static concepts; there are several steps in the research of quality:

1. Reference to a normative conventional treatment
2. Delivery of a perfect treatment
3. Reach excellency, gold standard
4. Creative innovation.

A. Mersel (✉)
Community Dentistry Hadassah School of Dental Medicine, University of Jerusalem, Jerusalem, Israel
e-mail: mersal@netvision.net.il

S. Carles
Dental & Oral Department, Faculty of Medicine and Health Sciences, School of Dentistry, Universitat de Barcelona, Barcelona, Spain
e-mail: subira@ub.edu

A. Mersel (ed.), *Treatment Dilemmas for Vulnerable Patients in Oral Health*,
https://doi.org/10.1007/978-3-031-08435-5_1

In our book, we will try to develop an Ethical approach in order to bring to the practitioner a simple, easy, and low-cost solutions for the handicapped and neglected patients.

In the last decades, Dental Profession has witnessed serious changes. The demographic status shows a huge increase in the elderly, socio-economic changes, and overall the technological revolution, influencing the patients' behavior.

Behavior changes are common with aging, and a permanent adaptation is necessary [1, 2].

As a result, there is a more important need and demand for oral and dental care. On the other hand, there are not enough practitioners and caregivers to deliver correct treatment to these neglected populations, including the old–old elderly, the handicapped children, and the special care adults. The ethical dilemmas are challenging from how to maintain a healthy aging population; how to face the chronic disease situations, how to manage the social and economic needs, and how to take care of the necessity of appropriate housing for long-term care. In several countries, there is a serious need of public policies.

Unfortunately, concerning the Oral Health aside the outstanding group of Gerontologists, very few programs was realized [3].

General Practitioners; GP have received in their Faculties very small instructions and post-graduate education in Geriatric Dentistry [4, 5].

In 2018 was published an expert opinion Policy with adapted Recommendations on Oral Health in Older Adults [5].

A survey realized in Belgium about the opinion of dentists on the barriers in providing oral care to frail older people underlined two main barriers: the lack of knowledge and the practical ignorance older people in Belgium [6].

Therefore, there is a real ethical dilemma between providing the "Best" care or to give a poor treatment and often no treatment at all. To face this problematic situation, the profession should understand that minimalistic intervention dentistry is necessary. In order to introduce such an approach, it is necessary to do a re-evaluation of the old educational dogmas [7].

Nevertheless, following a prodigious work, the educational situation is satisfactory in the USA where Geriatric Dentistry is required in 92.8% of the Dental Schools [8, 9].

MID, the Minimum Intervention Dentistry, is now providing some solutions for delicate ethical dilemmas. It is based on a changed approach in the management of the patients with priority to prevention and with a minimalistic intervention procedure [10].

Our book will discuss these issues.

2 The Demographic Dimension

The world population is constantly increasing. The WHO reported that the overall population over 60 years old will increase from 11% to 22% that means from 605 million in 2000 to 22 billion in 2050 (Fig. 1).

In Europe studies were trying to evaluate the prevalence and incidence of tooth loss in adult and elderly population [11].

In developing countries, this increase will occur strongly and will reach 1.7 billion in 2050. Another demographic trend will be the augmentation of the old–old population from 75 years old and over. This important group will present the most acute problems. This is a consequence of the ongoing decrease in the fertility and mortality decline of the elders. This evolution concerns the 65–75 years old group, the seniors, and also the 75–85 the old–old one. Also, the group of centenarians is even growing faster; estimated at 180,000 in 2000 and forecasted to one million in 2030. The median age indicates the age at which half of the population is older and the other half is younger. In the year 2000, the median age in the USA was 36 years twice the median age in Africa [12].

Another important factor is the retirement age. This social event was originally discussed

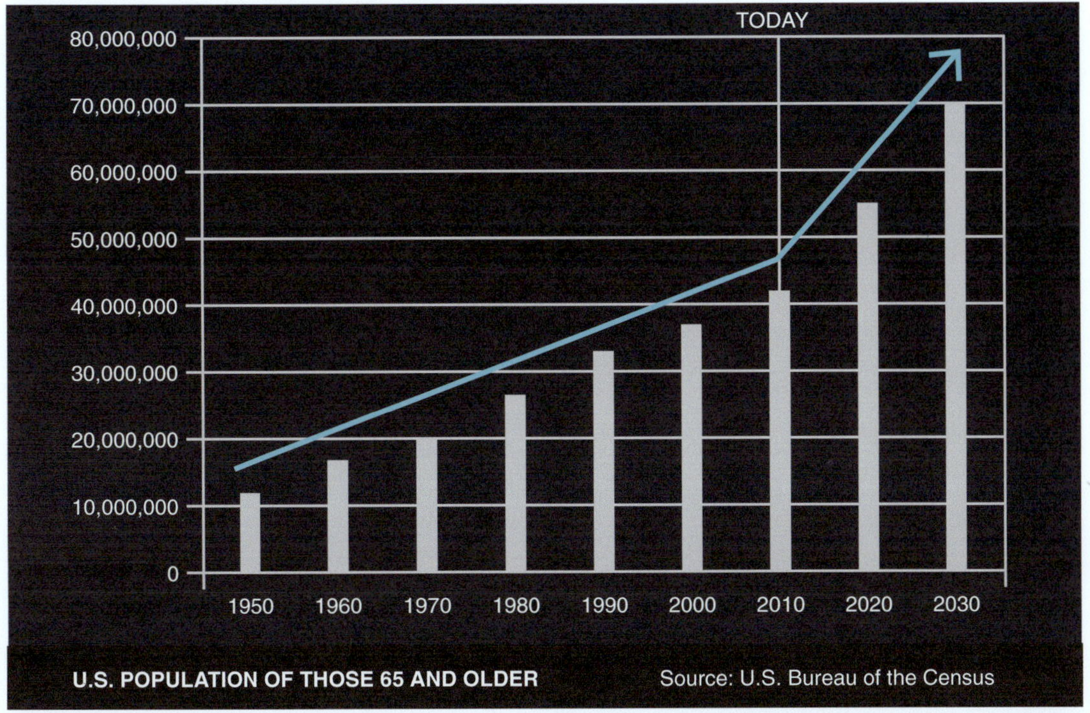

Fig. 1 Aging chart USA

by the German Canceler Bismarck (1884). After retirement, their social status changes and the elderly start depending on others. China, India, and Japan have the largest older population. In parallel, job-less people are in the same dependency burden group. In total, if one considers in the developed countries the number of the elderly (12–14%) and the number of unemployed persons (6–8%), we can summarize that about 20% of the population is facing difficulties on daily basis in order to survive. In addition to these facts, the estimations for the next decades point out a huge increase of the elders: 20–25% in 2030. Obviously, this will lead to an important percentage of neglected people (approximately 35%).

3 Socio-Economics Factors

After WW2, and the appearance of new economic standards and overall the high-tech supremacy in daily life, we witnessed a global transformation of the socio-economics structures. The concentration and urbanization of the inhabitants result in traffic jams and isolation of the individuals. Since that most of the women also are working very hard, the children are mainly alone. The lodgment crisis leads to smaller flats there is no place for a large family or the grandparents. The classical social and biological environment disappears. Since the school is not able to replace these structures, children play in the street neglecting their education and

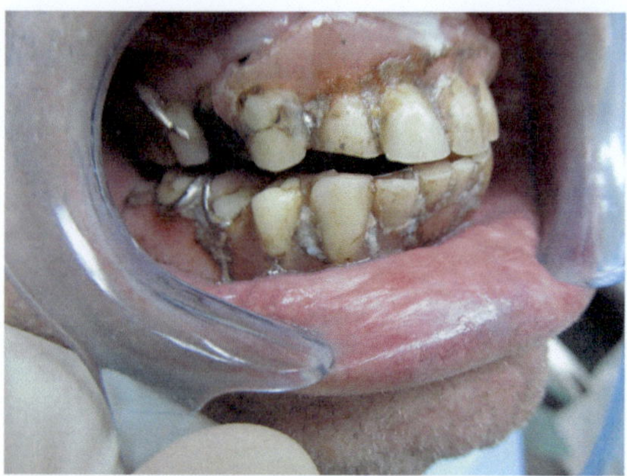

Fig. 2 Neglected right

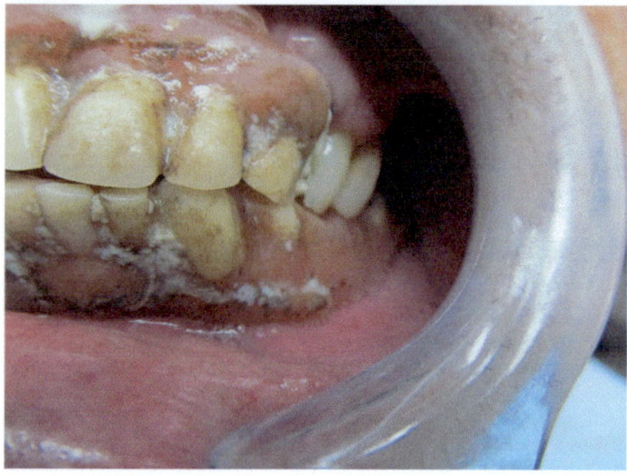

Fig. 3 Neglected left

Health, WHO and Nobel Biocare estimates (Figs. 2 and 3).

As mentioned, neglect is certainly a consequence of austerity but there are other factors as well [13].

3.1 Barriers to Treatment

There are a number of publications as a result of research for the reasons of the barriers to healthcare and lack of treatments for vulnerable patients.

3.1.1 The Time Factor

Emmanuel Kant, the great German philosopher, introduced transcendental notions of the space and the time. Space is well delimited and easily perceived element. Time is an ancestral notion divided in conjunction with astrological data; day and night hours and minutes. The watch is the conductor of the daily life.

But in fact, the value of the time is changing with the circumstances and the age. One hour for a young individual has not the same value as for an older or handicapped one. Therefore, we must take under consideration; the biological time, the psychological time, and the social time. Our patients need more time to understand, to remember, and to move, consequently; our timetable is not in harmony with their schedule and we have to modify our agenda. Ignoring this point will create anxiety, fatigue, and lead finally to the end of the treatment. Our patient will then join the huge group of neglected patients [14].

3.1.2 Mental or Psychological Evaluation

Psychiatry and Geriatrics are traditionally two different specialties. Nevertheless, mental illness makes a very important impact on each step of the treatment. It is obvious that a GP is not able to spend time and money learning these topics. It is also compulsory to understand very simple assessment for each patient. Therefore, it is recommended to be familiar with the main types of mental disorders to be present in the elderly or compromised people.

Dental Anxiety

Defined as distress or uneasiness of mind caused by fear of danger, this is a more relevant importantly to Phobia which is an irrational fear leading to an extreme desire to avoid the same painful situation. It was mentioned that dental anxiety is frequent in nearly of an half of the adult population [15].

Therefore, dental anxiety is a common barrier to oral care. The dentist should understand causes an effective management, capable of reducing anxiety and afterward the barriers to a high standard oral care [16].

Depression

There are different steps, but only patients at the early stage of this disease are coming for treatments. Depression in aging is common; surveys have indicated an incidence of about 15% for moderate to severe depression. In young patients, if life could be maintained, this disease eventually is expected to drive in the remission process. For elderly patients, depression will undermine the general health in the way that the remission when it comes will probably be too late. Before starting any treatment, a specified treatment is compulsory. The alert symptoms are anorexia, insomnia, self-neglected, loneliness, inertia, and overall the loss of motivation.

Organic Diseases

There are a large number of organic diseases that usually lead to chronic dementia which may be reversible after an appropriate treatment in the early stages. The clinical features are as follows:

- Some familiarity with the current events, but simple habits begin to deteriorate, difficulties to handle money.
- Confusion concerning the time, day, month, and year. Minor loss of memory.
- Behavior is reasonably appropriate but the patient has difficulty in choosing the "correct garment while dressing."
- Cannot give a rational response to a simple question.
- Obeys simple and clear commands. But the behavior may become sometimes antisocial.

Consequently, the dentist should, during the examination, run some assessment of the intellectual function; doing so he avoids during his treatment difficult situations such as the interruption of the treatment. In case of not following this practice will lead to a frustrated practitioner and to a neglected patient.

3.1.3 Medical Conditions and Risks Factors

Aging is not only pathology, but there is also a normal aging and pathologic diseases appearing with aging.

Basic "Normal" Aging Changes by Organs
- The Brain: Probability of decrease in brain weight/or the number of cells.

Increased atherosclerosis of cerebral vessels Lowliness.
- The Skin: Decreased response to pain, temperature, atrophy of the sweat glands, and loss of the subcutaneous fat padding.
- Arteries: Increased peripheral resistance and the diminution of elasticity and hypertension.
- Gastro-intestinal tract: Diminished hydrochloride and secretion. Decreased hepatic synthesis, and diminution of absorption of calcium.
- Renal: Diminution in size of the bladder. A decrease in the size of the kidneys and the number of glomeruli.
- Genital tract: Augmentation of the prostate gland. Decrease in vaginal and cervical secretions, but not the total end of the sexual function.
- Musculoskeletal systems: Diminution of the muscle size and function. Decreased synthesis and degradation of the bone.
- Eye: Difficulties for accommodation, increased density of the lens, loss of elasticity of the lens, and change of the aqueous kinetics.
- Ears: Anatomical changes in the inner ear and in the cochlea.
- Heart: Decreased cardiac muscle, increased valves calcification, and sclerosis of the conduction system.
- Lungs: Increased size of the alveoli, and decreased diffusion and surface area across the alveolar–capillary membrane.
- Immunological status: Deceased cell T function.
- Hormones: Deceased metabolic clearance, estrogen, and deceased insulin peripheral response.

During the first interview and history taking, it is necessary for the dentist to establish personal timing and duration in order to deal with the chief complaint before they started.

3.1.4 Medical Advises

Frequently, there is a simultaneous coexistence and interdependence of several diseases in contrary to the younger patients. Often the patients and also the family hide the medical status of the patient.

It seems clear that aging appears to be the most important risk factor for the deterioration of normal physiological functions, and the main organ-specific pathologies.

The dentist must be aware that; there is an illness with long latent periods; there are age-related diseases and a decline of the immune function. Falls are frequent; women fall more than men.

- Diabetes mellitus is an important cause of morbidity and mortality in old age. The incidence rises with the age with a prevalence of 3% for over 65 year's age. The majority are obese and non-insulin dependent.
  Diabetes leads to a number of complications such as:
  Vascular and cerebrovascular diseases, renal failures, formation of premature cataract and retinopathies, and other infections. The dentist should take special care before starting an invasive procedure [17].
- Cerebrovascular disease
  A stroke is the consequence of a sudden interruption of the blood flow and is the third major killer and the direct cause of disability. The incidence of strokes is increasing with aging, hypertension, obesity, and hyper-glycemia.
- Parkinson's disease has become very prevalent with the longevity increase, now being the second most important neurodegenerative disorder in the world [18].
- Cancer
  Aging is one of the major factors determining this disease. There are several reasons:
  - Cariogenesis could be stimulated by changes in the hormonal control.
  - Immunological mechanism might fall with aging.
  - A longer life allows a longer exposure to environmental factors.

For geriatric patients, a great majority of cancer occurred in the lungs, the skin, the breast, stomach, and the prostate [19] (Fig. 4).

The Mouth; the fact that over a half of the elder patients have not considered consulting a dentist for about 10 years explained this neglected situation of the mouth; not only the teeth and the dentures, but also the tongue, the lips, and the jaws.

Usually, there is a remarkable absence of pain. Cancer is more frequent in women than in men, but the dentist must also be aware that there are manifestations in a younger age.

During the first consultation, an acute examination is mandatory and from an ethical point of view, it should be under the responsibility of the practitioner.

- Organic brain syndromes: Dementia Alzheimer; AD and SDAT. Alzheimer is associated with two characteristic pathologic changes with dementia starting in pre-senile age; senile plaques and intra-neuronal neurofibrillary tangles in AD, above 65 years of age, are the characteristics of SDAT.

Research studies have shown that 5–6% of the elderly have organic dementia.

The dentist must be aware that this illness has an insidious onset, and is progressing step by step to the final stage. Intellectual deficit dominate the main functions; reduction of memory and language, disorientation, time confusion, and visual-spatial recognition.

The emotional state is presenting agitation, disturbances, aggressiveness, and stress intolerance. Since this important pathology starts slowly without dramatic symptoms, the patient and his family ignore this fact. Therefore, treatment starts easily, but if the treatment plan is scheduled for a long time, the end could be dramatic. The treatment will be interrupted and the patient will be neglected (Fig. 5).

Fatigue is one of the features characterizing the frailty syndrome, compromising the normal development of therapeutic planning [20].

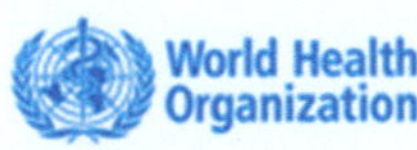
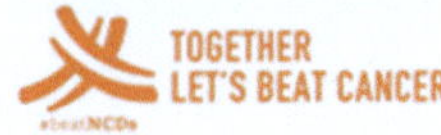

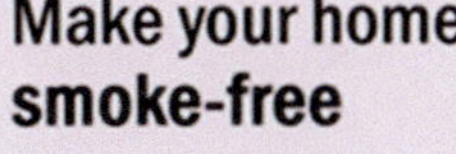

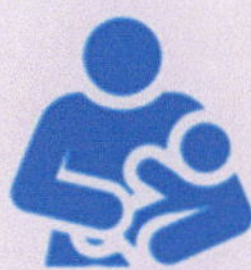

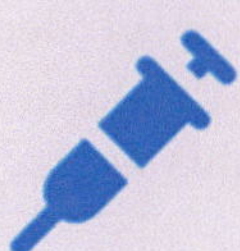

Fig. 4 Cancer prevention

- Polypharmacy
  The proportion of elders taking drugs is 80–95% [21].
  In comparison to 30% with younger people aged from 20 to 65. There are several factors influencing drug behavior:
  - The great number of different drugs
  - The number of doses prescribed for each individual
  - The errors and the omissions
  - During the investigation, patients do not remember the name of their drugs.
  - As a consequence, the dentist is not able to start the treatment until this fact is not resolved.

3.1.5 The Economic Background

- Financial Conditions: The income of the elderly population is in average less than the younger population.
  In the last decade, it was difficult to maintain financial security for the aging population. Obviously, fixed incomes cannot keep up with the inflation rate. In the USA, around 25% are close to the poverty level.

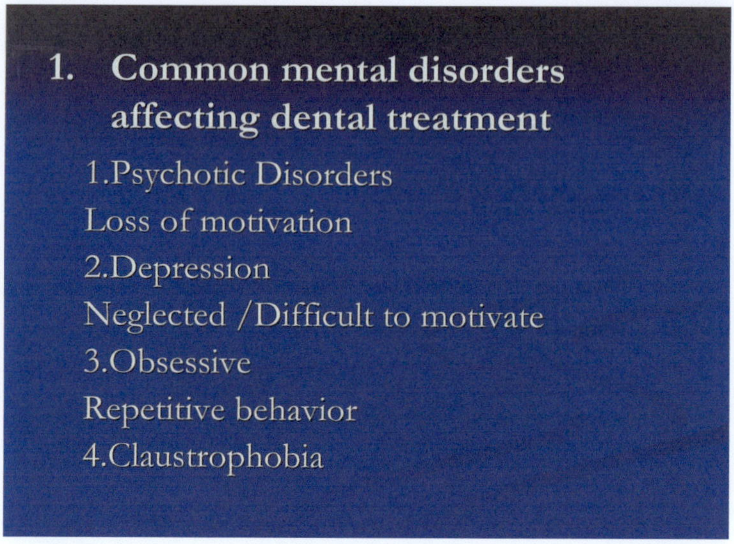

Fig. 5 Assistance

> **1. Common mental disorders affecting dental treatment**
> 1.Psychotic Disorders
> Loss of motivation
> 2.Depression
> Neglected /Difficult to motivate
> 3.Obsessive
> Repetitive behavior
> 4.Claustrophobia

Furthermore, elderly living alone with no relative have a very low income. Sometimes at retirement, the income drops down to 50%. In general, it is probably possible that the economic needs of this population are less than those of the young population but certainly, their needs are decreased by half at their retirement.

In North Europe, according to Ferrera's welfare typology, the medical and socio-economic situation seems to be more favorable.

The oral health and welfare state regimes were analyzed by a cross-national report about of European countries [22].

In 2005, already Erik Petersen Head of WHO's Oral Health Program stated that: unless we take action today, many countries will not be able to pay for dental treatment.

Bulletin of the WHO [23].

- Living condition: A majority of the elderly is living in a family with the spouse (75%), others live alone (10%), and a smaller proportion (15%) lives in nursing homes or institutions.

Two-thirds are living in urban central cities or small towns.

Often the children and friends live too far and the elders are left without social and financial support. Elders are concentrated in a nice climate area as in the state of Florida; other six other states contain a half of the US elders.

- Health Insurances: The expenses for healthcare are constantly increasing. Because of the new technologies, the cost of dental treatment is very high, which does not allow a correct treatment for this neglected group.

Because of this fact we are witness of a number of national or Individual insurances (art. assur). In European countries and other developed nations, there are national systems offering financing the expenses by act or by capita.

Nevertheless, this procedure obliged the practitioner to submit the treatment plan and other medical acts to prior authorization.

In addition, this classical insurance contracts allows for each individual the reimbursement of the treatments; partially or totally.

When a total restoration is necessary people cannot afford it, therefore only a small part of the treatment is realized leaving the patients in a neglected situation.

3.1.6 The Distance and the Accessibility of the Clinics

In addition to the elderly living in nursing homes or community houses, a number of elders are staying in their old apartments or residences. Consequently, they are consulting the same clinic for a long time. Unfortunately, what was easy is now very difficult; the distance remains the same but the track is not yet possible. Usually dental clinics have no good access for wheel chairs even others are located in higher flats without an elevator. Therefore, when there is no organized transportation, these people become neglected patients.

Cees de Baat: 3A: Availability, Affordability, and Acceptability.

Defined by The 3A's access process [24].

3.1.7 The Lack of Adequate Equipment

Practitioners need to invest in their equipment. Since modern technologies had changed the design of the dental office few offices are offering these services to handicapped people. Another point is the Rural–Urban differences in Dentist supply.

One of the major causes of oral heath diseases is the lack of access to dental services. In a survey done in Kentucky, it was found that out of 120 countries, 42 had shortage in dental supply [25].

3.1.8 Insufficient Working Force

The last demographic estimation show that there will be serious increase of elderly people was accurate. The percentage of the elderly in Germany is 20.4%, UK is 20.7%, France is 19.3%, Italy is 20.6%, and Spain is 18.9% (Table 1).

Also in Africa, the population is aging; 11.9% of the African population is older than 60 years; about 25 million [26].

There are not enough dentist and auxiliaries teams to fulfill the charges of a minimalistic oral health service.

The majority (52%) of care homes visited had no policy to promote and protect oral health. Nearly half (47%) of the homes are not providing any staff training. Almost 73% of the resident's care plans reviewed did not cover Oral health … as stated by the Care Quality Commission. Dentistry.

3.1.9 Inadequate Training and Skill of the Dental Team

Providing oral health care for elderly and special patients is the aim for practitioners trained for this challenge.

For the elderly, Geriatric Dentistry or Gerodontology is the name of the Specialty dealing with the universities dental faculties or Schools. We come to the conclusion that in general, Gerodontology is not taught in every institution. Concerning post-dental education, Gerodontology is not often a part of the official syllabus. The duration of the training and the content of the dental education curriculum vary. Geriatric dentistry has not been established as a standalone course in the majority of countries, with the exception of Japan. There is a lack of dentists trained in geriatric dentistry as well as training programs [27].

In an expert Opinion from the European College of Gerodontology, it was mentioned that one of the barriers is the lack of professional support including limited training in caring frail and care-dependent elders, and also the poor knowledge of oral health providers? [28].

In a survey concerning Higher Education in European Universities it was concluded:

- That a large proportion of Dental Schools (82%) teach Gerodontology at the undergraduate level that means by only classical educational systems without any clinical support.
- In the same way, postgraduate geriatric dentistry education is included in several of the Specialties Programs since Gerodontology is not recognized as a normal specialty [29].
- When an official and mandatory continuing education exists, very few are devoted to this issue.
- Moreover, in these disciplines, practical hands-on is compulsory to reach a convenient skill. Nevertheless, in the last decade, an outstanding effort was done by the European Gerontologist.

Table 1 Life expectancy and healthy life expectancy by economic status (2012)

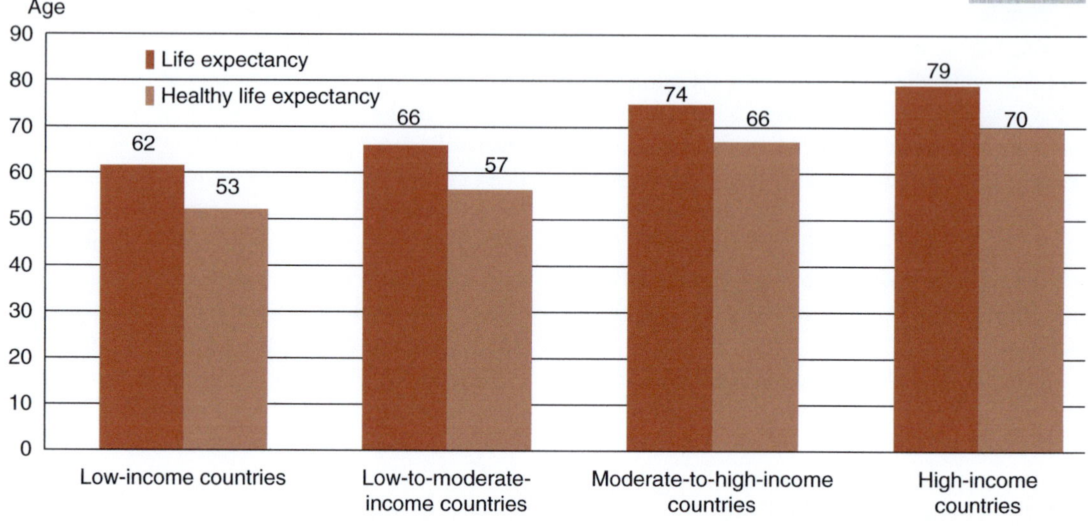

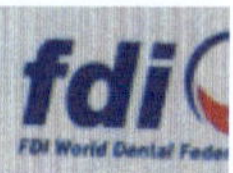

Source: WHO World Health Statistics 2014

All these authors concluded that there is an urgent need in revising the education system.

In the USA, RL. Ettinger started to establish a separate and specialized concept in Geriatric dentistry. In 1996, with a group of pioneers an article was published: The old–old dental patient: the Challenge of clinical decision making a loss of collaboration and planning with the authorities [30].

In the FDI Europe regional Continuing Education Program, two separated surveys were realized:

1. Yamalik, N. Mersel, A, were starting a Survey and Analysis of the extent and efficiency of the partnership and collaboration between the dental faculties and the National Dental Associations within the FDI-ERO zone:

   This survey had an aim to discover the attitudes of the Faculties toward cooperation with the NDA's. The findings pointed out that there is not a positive trend for close cooperation. It even can be said that dental faculties and NDA's sometimes act as two different organizations.

2. Afterwards a second research examined the Collaboration between dental Faculties and national dental associations within the World Dental Association, FDI – European Regional Association; NDS' Perspective. The aim of this study was to evaluate the areas of collaboration between the NDAs and the dental faculties. The present study highlighted the importance of an active cooperation between the two organizations. In the majority (63%), the NDAs felt that counterparts treated each other as a partner, except some NDAs who stated that areal was not evident. Therefore, there is a need to improve a regular and efficient partnership [31].

3.1.10 A Little Motivation from the Professional Organizations

FDI Policy Statement 1997 Seoul. International Principles of Ethics for the Dental Profession. Only one simple point the Dentist "must deal ethically in all aspects of professional life and adhere to the rules of professional law."

"An Alarm rose over oral health of elderly Brits." According to the new report published by the Royal College of Surgeons, eight million of over ten million live with dental pain, oral sepsis, or extensive caries and untreated teeth.

In Canada a survey find out severe Inequity in the Oral Health Care for Elderly Canadians. Provoking ethical dilemmas [32].

The study points out that 53% of elder patients do not possess a dental insurance at all.

2016: FDI Project for Oral Health for ageing population World Oral Health Forum establishment of a Road map concerning three essential points:

1. Investigations effective measures of prevention.
2. Investigations between the linkage of oral health and general health.
3. To close the health gap reducing barriers in access to oral health care "we need to study and identify the most effective ways to target the social determinants of Oral Health."

3.1.11 An In-Depth Look at Oral Health and Healthy Aging

The dental profession could not find practical solutions for acute problems in daily practice [33] (Fig. 6).

2018: An expert opinion from the European College of Gerodontology and the European Geriatric Medicine Society proposed recommendations on Oral Health in Older Adults; three major areas were identified:

1. Education for healthcare providers
2. Health policy actions
3. Citizens' empowerment and involvement.

In conclusion, since the profession is challenging, the education track is the most recommended track [34].

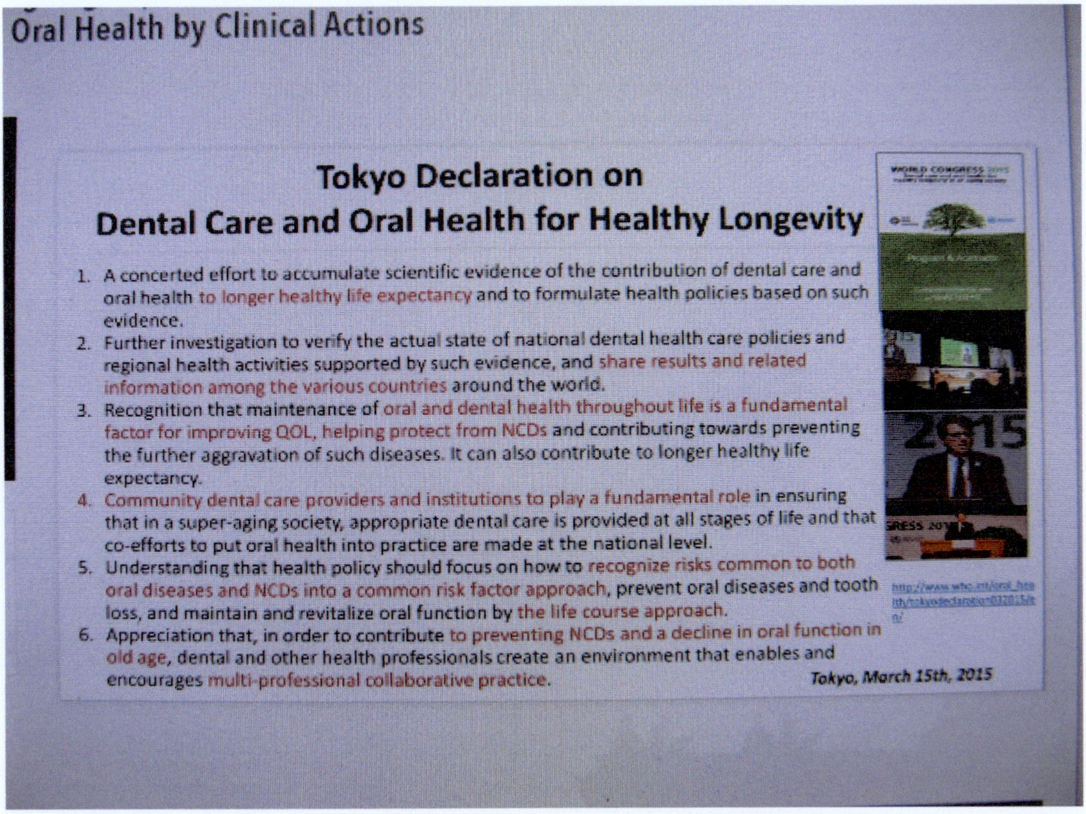

Fig. 6 Tokyo declaration

3.1.12 Continuing Education; Variable Collaboration with the Faculties and the Universities

The association for Dental Education in Europe and the EU Commission has adopted a directive for the recognition of professional qualities. Concerning Gerodontology, this educational process is variable. These range from well-established courses to very little being readily identified in the curriculum. Sometimes surprisingly the deans do not want the little that was already included. This is the result of complex relationship between different authorities.

The real problem is not the syllabus in Geriatric Dentistry but the content and the practical skill; there are too much theories and not enough clinical training [35].

Globally, there are TWO parallel structures:

- The universities are in charge of the undergraduate and postgraduate education.
- The professional organizations such as National Dental Associations, Dental Chambers, Private Institutions are supporting the whishes and the claims of the Dental community in several aspects and particularly in continuing education. As the profession is dealing with continuous challenges; maintaining the scientific level in this way is the guarantee of the quality of the treatments [36].

Since this is finally also a public health concern, each country is deciding which structures will run the Continuing Education System. Consequently, political aspects are inserted and each country in Europe is ruled by the Council of European Dentists dependent on the EU Council: Code of Ethics for Dentists in the European Union.

4 Evaluation and Evolution in Continuing Education

Usually continuing education is monitored by several tracks, congresses, courses, seminars, e-learning, and videos. Continuing education can be voluntary or compulsory. In major European countries, obligatory programs are present for all active dentists.

There is a progressive evolution of the continuing education **programs** in Europe. The Speakers are now more aware about the specificity teaching to adult and experimented colleagues [37].

A trustful evaluation is the sound basis of an attempt for an adapted evolution. Studies showed a gap between the education programs and what the general practitioner will like to learn. This influences, of course, the satisfaction of the participants (Table 2).

Table 2 Desirata … wishes for the future

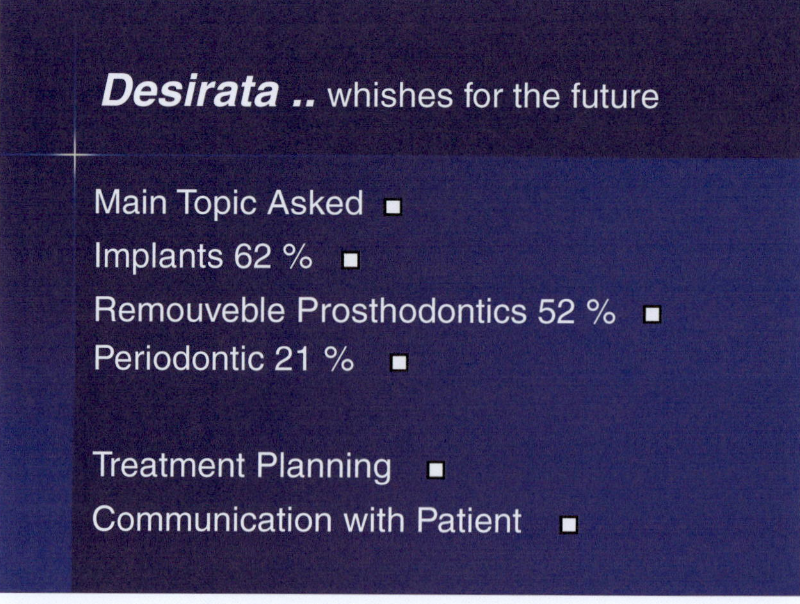

The actual evaluation is mainly managed by questionnaires which the public is not enthusiastic to fulfill. Therefore, an appropriate system was launched and in parallel with a specific preparation of the speakers. A good scientific researcher is not necessarily a good lecturer.

There is no doubt that the new technology will have a tremendous influence for our profession in the future. However, our major ethical challenge is to develop an adapted approach toward the neglected groups. To realize this evolution, it is imperative to set up a realistic evaluation system.

5 Ethical Concerns for Oral Health

Oral Health in a state of crisis, says Lancet. Is this true or exaggerated? What is obvious is that extreme Oral Health inequalities exist for the most marginalized and socially excluded group; the neglected patients.

The profession has the heavy duty to face this Ethical dilemma. In 2007, appeared the booklet edited by the FDI entitled: Dental Ethics manual; which was distributed to all the National Dental Association. Another book entitled: Ethical considerations for the Oral healthcare of frail elders, was published by Blackwell in 2011 and edited by Michael L. MacEntee In order to clarify the situation, some points are important.

For a long time, the notion of ethics appeared in the Medical profession; from Hippocrates to Maimonides to the actual recommendations. Ethics do not represent a code of Law, not an Obedience, not only a feeling, not a habit, and not only a consensus. Deontology is defined as a basis for making moral decisions, but once the rules are established, they have to be implementing in specific conditions. The three main principles of our profession are as follows:

1. To practice according to the science of Dentistry
2. To respect the principles of Humanity
3. To safeguard the Oral Health of the patients without any individual restrictions.

The WHO and the official authorities took the responsibility of realizing these aims. Unfortunately, despite valuable effort, the profession is far from a solution. Consequently, there is a need for a new concept, the **Consequentialisms**.

An ethical decision making based on the consequences and outcomes of different choices and procedures will lead to utilitarianism using "utility" as a measure and the definition "the greatest good for the greatest number."

In fact, doing some is better than doing nothing. Neglected persons are looking desperately for help. Reviewing the planning strategies will adopt simple procedures in order to investigate the immediate needs.

In this way, Virtue Ethics will allow by accepting minimum standards for maximal care. Very eminent scientific and leading personalities have already launched adapted concepts.

Education by the creation of a new ethical environment will allow the optimal care for handicapped patients. In this way, the dentist should consider the patient's best interests on priority [38].

5.1 Code of Ethics for Dentists in the European Union. 2007. President

From the clinical aspects, a number of questions appear. Will our treatment reduce the patient's pain or discomfort? Are you taking risks? Will it improve the quality of life? What is the physiological and psychological background? Is there a liable communication with patients and his family? An appropriate ethical decision making in aged care might be difficult and time-consuming, and often the success depends about the socio-economic influences. The dentists influence the Oral Health of their patients; therefore, ethics must be their guidelines (Fig. 7).

Fig. 7 Top work ethics

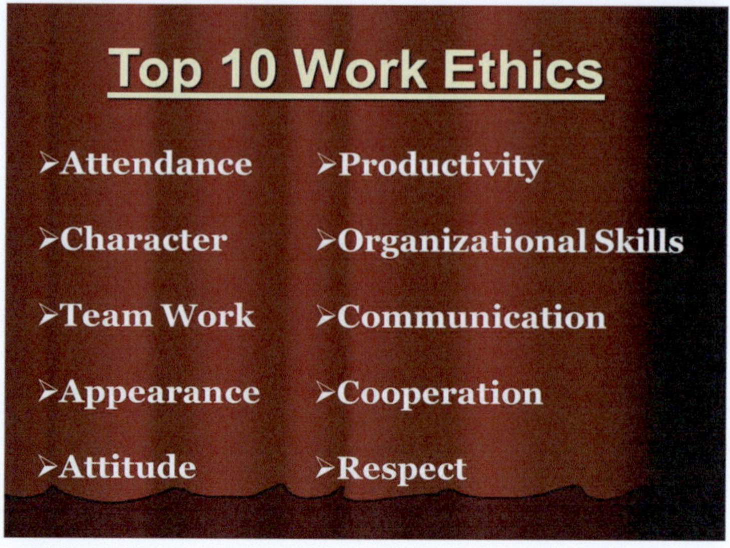

6 Approaches for Clinical Solutions

6.1 The Dogmas Obstacle

In general, the dentists receive an excellent education concerning the basic disciplines. Despite the fact that they apply the rules they were taught, they are often disappointed with the results. Unfortunately, some classical dogma is dragging down the clinical procedures to the pitfall. As Claude Bernard said, "It is what we think we know already, that often prevents us from learning."

Step by step, we witness the silent conflict between the classic conventional teaching and a more adapted clinical approach [39].

The crucial problems for an adapted occlusion are an important reason for many failures; a bilateral articulation might bring the solution [40].

The patient's satisfaction with complete dentures: obviously do not depend on technical updates, but often in the patient personality [41].

Nevertheless, conventional education is strongly maintained by the faculties and also by the publication of books presenting the same schemas. Hereby a short approximatively list is provided:

- *Complete Dentures: Swenson by Mosby 1940*
- *Prosthodontic Treatment: Boucher by Mosby 1975*
- *Designing Complete Dentures: Watt and MacGregor by Saunders 1976*
- *Dental care of the elderly Atlas: Drummond, Newton, Yemm by Mosby Wolfe 1995*
- *Prosthodontics for the Elderly: Budtz-Juergensen by Quintessence Books 1999*
- *The Complete Denture; A clinical Pathway: MacEntee by Quintessence book 2nd Edition 2014.*

The satisfaction of patients about their oral restoration is a key factor concerning the success of their treatment. Unfortunately as a result of poor clinical quality, patients' feedback is not appropriate. In a comparison of 500 Patients about their appreciation of the quality of their Dentures: as a result of the failure, these patients are classified as part of the neglected group.

6.2 The New Trends

Since the last few decades, in different specialties, we witness an evidence-based evolution.

In a survey Prof. Yamalik, N. had checked the implementation of evidence-based dentistry (EBD) into practice; analysis of awareness, perceptions, and attitudes of dentists in the World Dental Federation—Europe Regional

Organization zone. A few number of countries (32.1%) adapted this relatively new concept [42].

A. Classic Prosthodontics: Locking on the theories based procedures, there was actually a new approach, and hereby some examples are given.

6.2.1 Complete Dentures

Impressions. Phonetic impressions, Registration of the Neutral zone, Dynamic Registration of the Tongue's movements and Piezography which is the impression of the inner and outer walls of the Prosthetic corridor, or the Prosthetic physiological Space.

The main Authors were [43–45]:

- *Beresin, V. Shiesser, F. The Neutral zone in complete dentures. Book Second Edition. 1978. C. V. Mosby Ed. Saint Louis.*
- *Klein, P. Prothese Piezographique; Prothese totale adjointe geriatrique. Ed. John Libbey 1988. ISBN 0-86196-141-2.*
- *Mersel A. Gerodontology – A contemporary Prosthetic Challenge Part-1: Mandibular Impression Technique. 1987. Gerodontology 6-1: 79–81.*
- *Harster, P. Tissue Modeling: the Oral pump. Quintessence International. 2005; 36: 633–640.*
- *Mersel, A. and Eisenberg. Dental Asia. Physiological Design of the complete denture space. 2012. 11–12: 24–26.*
- *With the introduction of the CAD/CAM, the utilization of this technique was recently witnessed for the realization of impressions in complete denture. If this procedure might be acceptable for an anatomic one, for a functional impression, this system is not valuable for the registration of physiological movements.*
- *Srinivasan, M. and all. CAD/CAM milled removable complete dentures: an in vitro evaluation of trueness [46].*
- *Goodacre, C.J. and all. 2012. CAD/CAM fabricated complete denture concepts and clinical methods of obtaining required morphological data. J of Prosthetic Dentistry. 1: 1–10 [47].*

- *Moreover this method is not able to register and transfer the different pressure on the soft issues; a crucial step in the Impressions stage.*

6.2.2 Jaw Relations Records: Occlusion for Edentulous Patients

Occlusion remains one of the most important issues in oral restoration or more exactly rehabilitation. Concerning this challenge, we have to take into consideration the multiple and fundamental functions of the mouth; esthetics, speech, mastication, swallowing, and sexuality. Physiological swallowing functions deteriorate with aging, even in dentate persons, but the masticatory system remains the key target.

Authors—Between the numerous pioneers:

Alfred Gysi and J. Leon Williams 1910–1914 on an artificial tooth system. Ulf Posselt: Physiology of Occlusion and Rehabilitation. Blackwell Ed. 1962. Bonwill, Benett, and Snow on Kinesiology of the occlusion. Thielemann and Hanau on the articulation forma. Their studies drawn down to registration of the inter-maxillary relationship, then to dynamics of the mastication and finally, the transmission of the different factors to an articulator. At this time, the dental profession was witnessing real articulator wars.

Actually, it is to be noted that there are two main types; fully adjustable and semi-adjustable articulators. Usually, the general practitioner and the dental technician operate with a simplified model (Figs. 8 and 9).

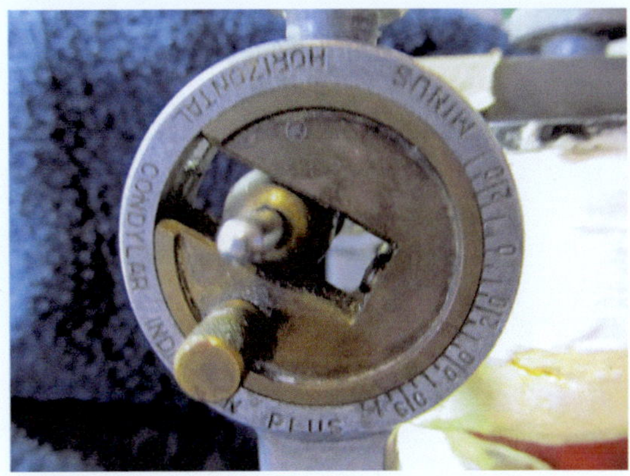

Fig. 8 Condylar guidance

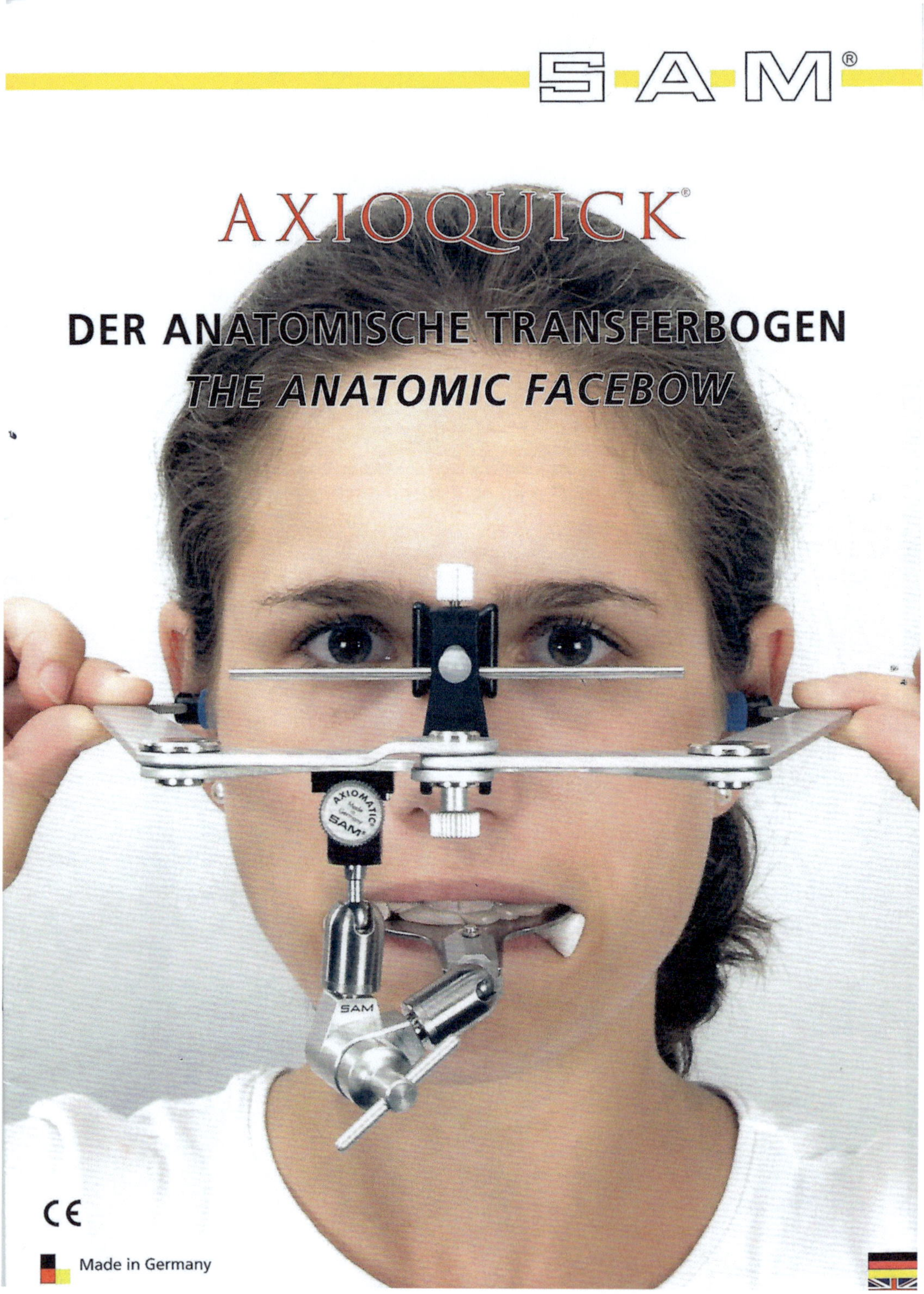

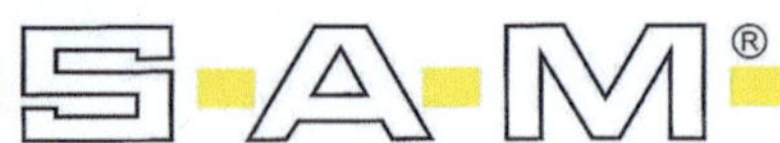

Fig. 9 Face-bow

6.2.3 Limits of the Conventional Systems

Numerous practitioners are surprised by the fact that despite the conventional laws were perfectly realized, a great number of their patients were not satisfied. To avoid break down during the treatment, elaborating the treatment planning a qualitative investigations are compulsory … [48].

Scientific laws are based on universal laws but with time, some important changes appear. For example, the axiom that posterior teeth must be situated on the residual crest, this might be exact for young seniors, but what is the situation for the old–old group. With the continual changes of the anatomic and physiologic landmarks new intermaxillary relations appear requesting personal teeth set up for each patient [49, 50].

Looking in the old literature, we find that the figures dealt with individuals aged 45–50 years old. From the Book of Victor H. Sears [51] (Figs. 10 and 11).

The same remark is valuable for the Hinge axis location, the vertical dimension, and the occlusal orientation plane. The fundamental principle is that all the patients are **different**; therefore, looking for a symmetric approach is the Dentist responsibility and does not make sense.

There is a growing minority of atypical or unusual persons looking for prosthodontics that presents outstanding features or variations from the "normality," and who are unable to receive conventional treatment, or cannot wear the dentures suggested by their dentist. In fact, as a result, this group becomes a part of the neglected patients [52].

6.3 Neutral Zone and Phonetic Impressions

The conventional impression techniques often ignore important factors as the tongue and the design of the dentures. The tongue during function interferes with the polished acrylic form of the denture. The registration of the neutral zone will help realize a harmonious contact with the peripheral structures. The neutral zone impression technique or Piezography is a noninvasive and quick procedure, allowing a harmonious

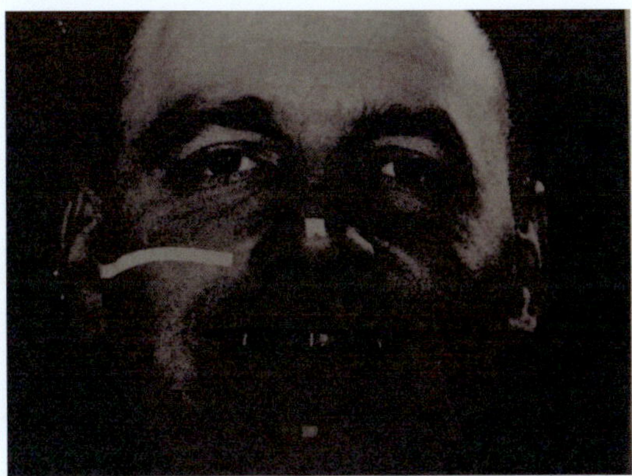

Fig. 10 Book photo men; Swenson Ed, 1940

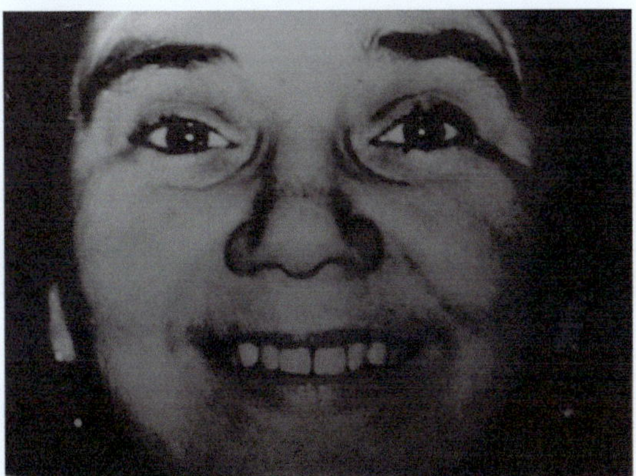

Fig. 11 Book photo women

adaptation of the lower denture. The Mandibular restoration seems to be the major obstacle for a physiologic rehabilitation, as the consequence of the ignorance about the tongue, and the relationship of the tongue and the Phonetics [53, 54] (Figs. 12, 13, 14, 15, 16, 17, 18, 19, and 20).

The determination of a correct Plane of occlusion, the respect of the Neutral zone are the imperative conditions of a physiological insertion of the complete dentures [55, 56].

6.4 Establishment of the Plan of Occlusion

After the registration of the vertical dimension and before the determination of the centric relation, dentist is obliged to fix the occlusal plane.

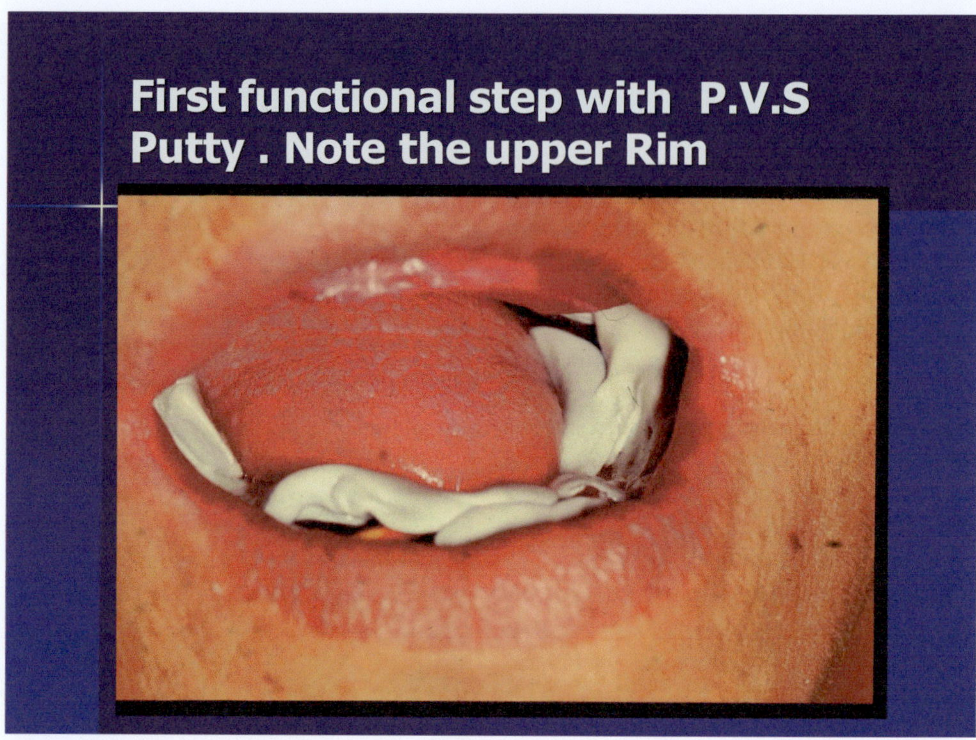

Fig. 12 Functional impression first step

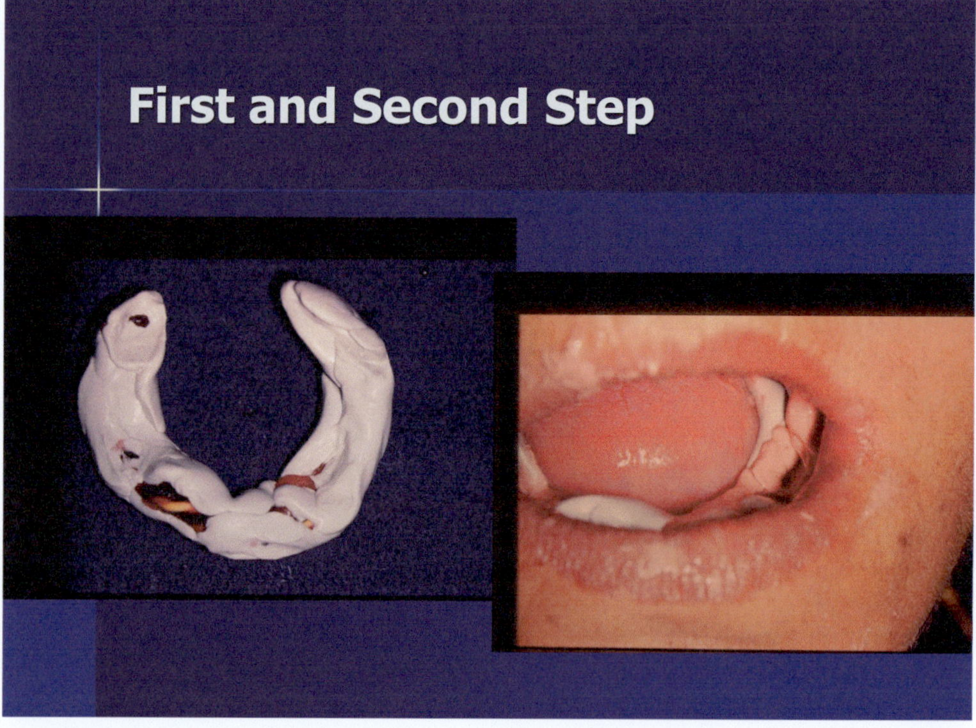

Fig. 13 Functional impression second step

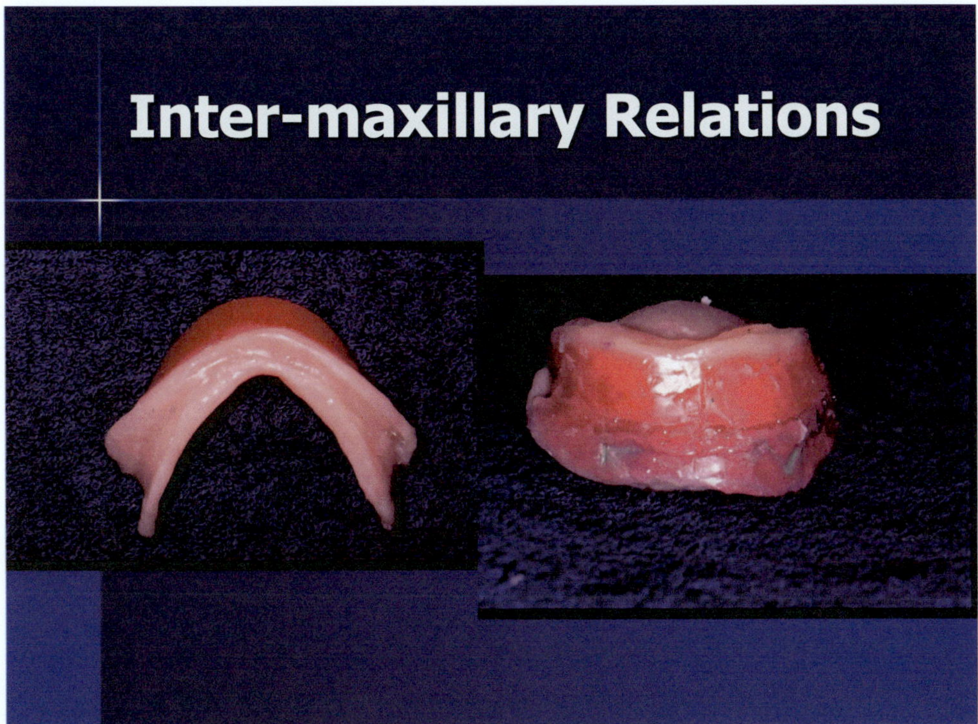

Fig. 14 Intermaxillary relationship

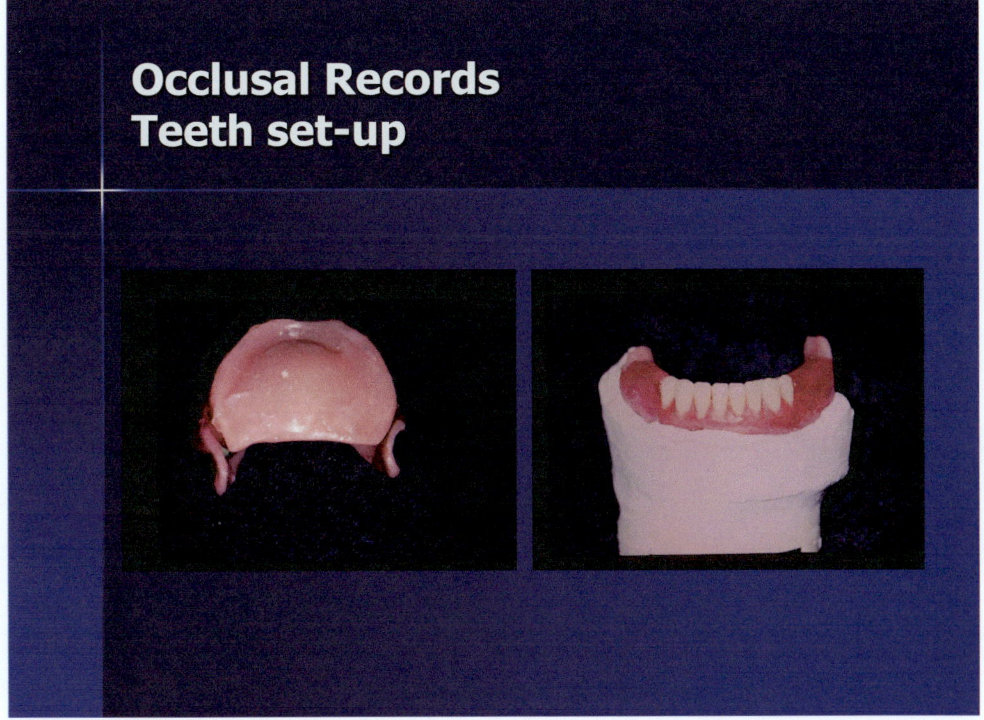

Fig. 15 Occlusal records—teeth set up

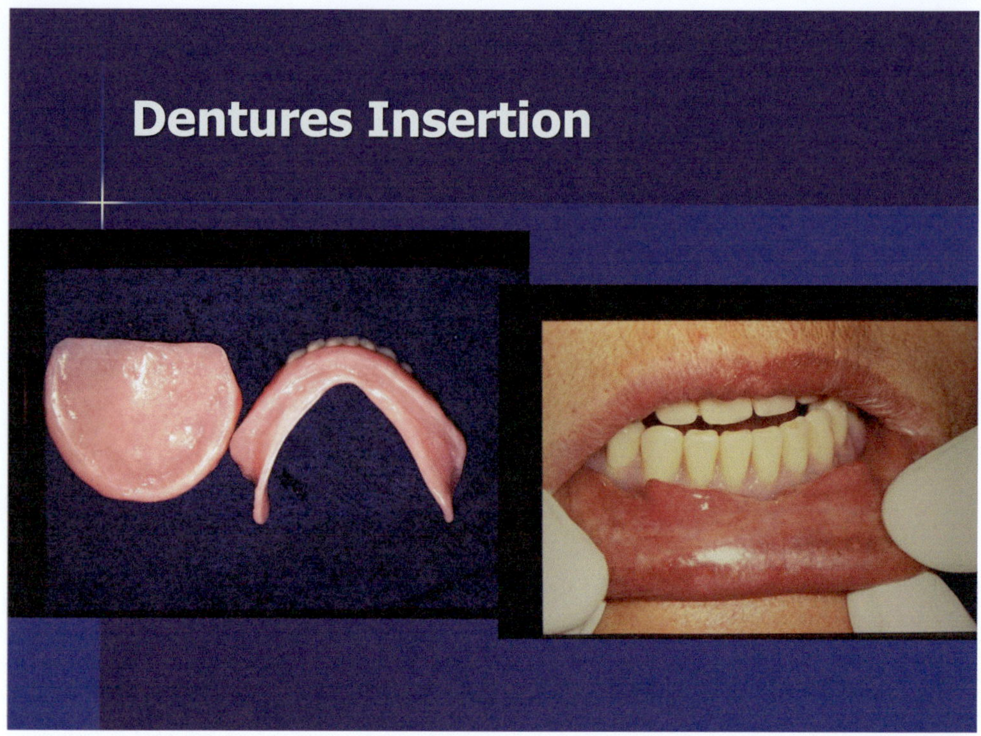

Fig. 16 Dentures insertion

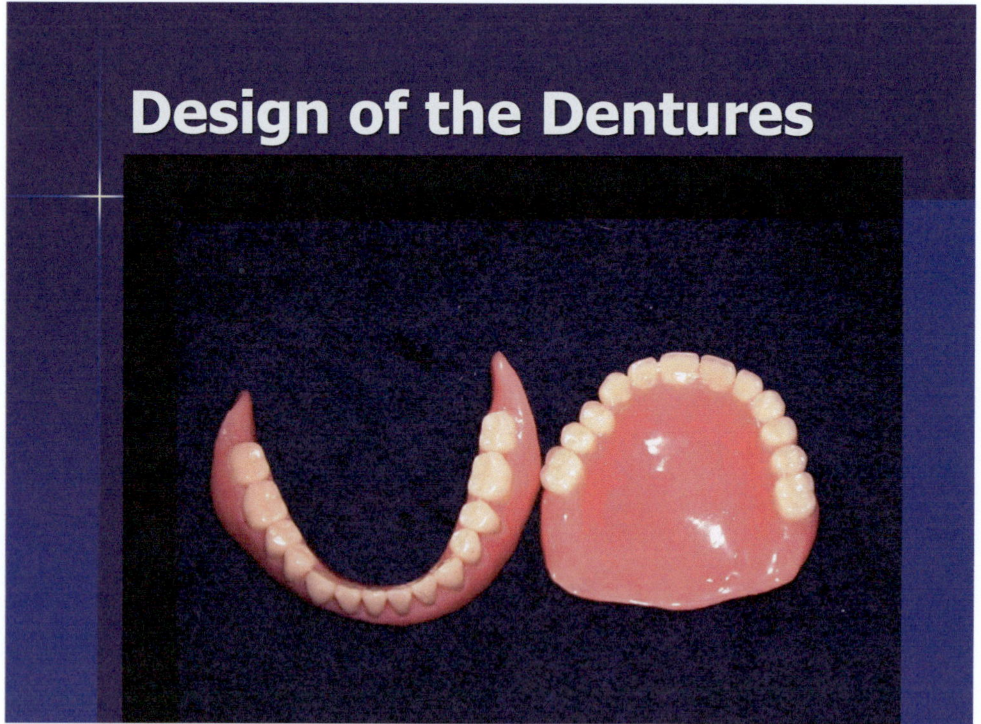

Fig. 17 Design of the dentures

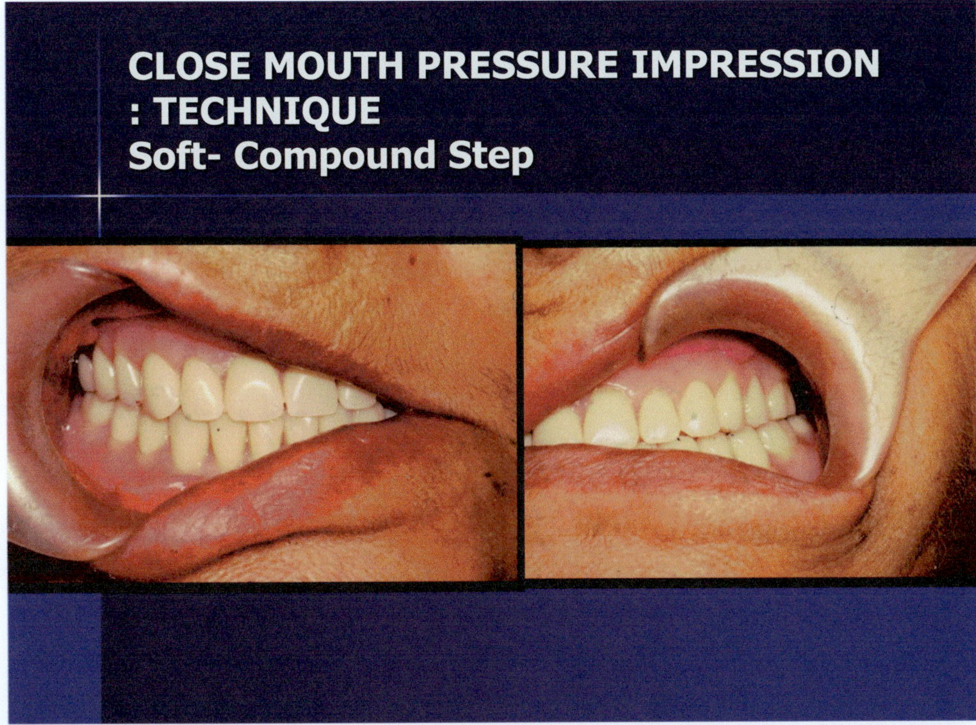

Fig. 18 Close mouth pressure impression

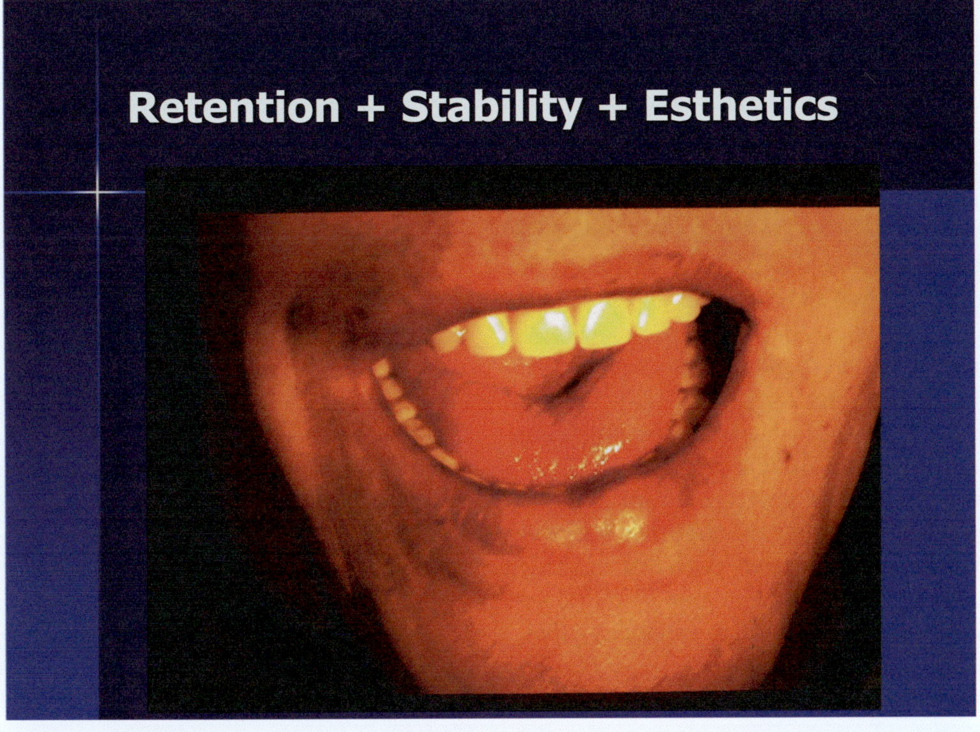

Fig. 19 Retention and stability

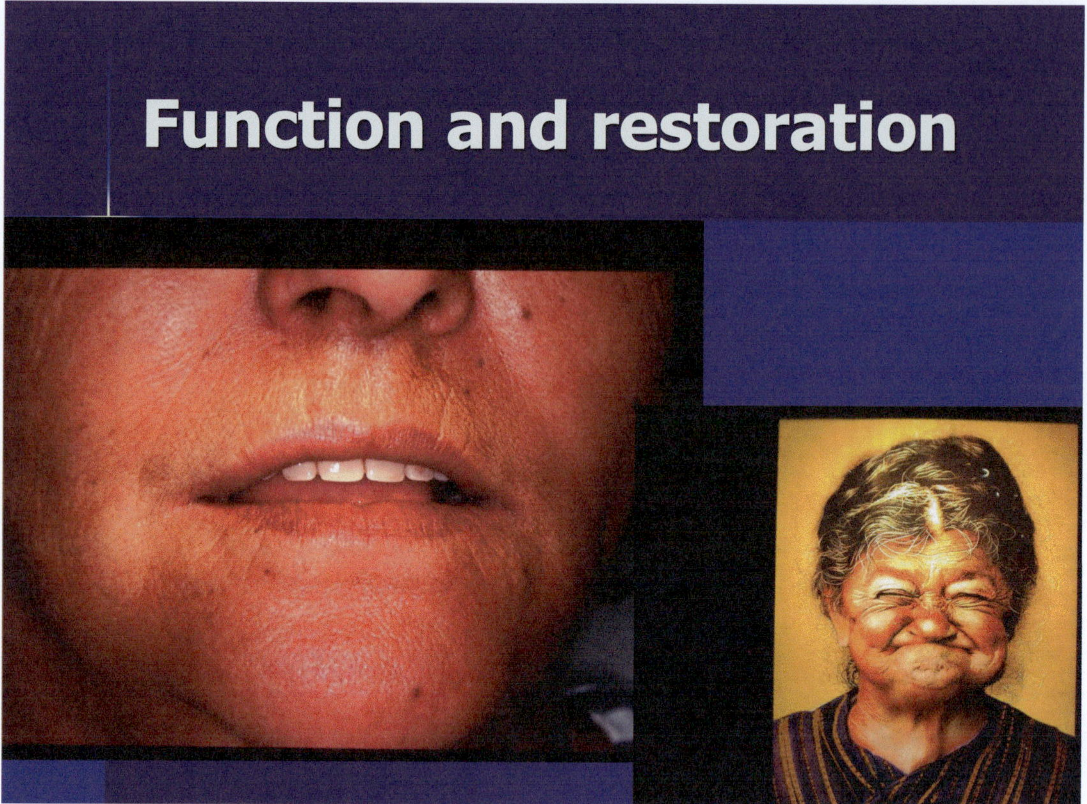

Fig. 20 Piezography and esthetics

There is often confusion in this step as some use the Frankfort Horizontal Plane for reference; and the result will be a premature contact with the posterior segment and a gliding a dislodging of the mandibular denture.

Others are using the camper plane as a reference. The Camper was a Dutch anatomist, and his plane referred only to: "the upper skeletal" anatomy. There is no consideration about the tongue, a vital and dynamic organ, and the mandibular denture (Fig. 21).

In order to overrule these problems, researchers started to find a novel approach.

Prof. Chalapathi Rao inclined plane effect and leverage in the meantime, another group was working on a new trend which involved first: creating a mandibular design by registration of the tongue phonetic movements and the peripheral envelope.

Second, taking advantage of this phonetic impression, a mandibular <u>occlusal plane is established</u> (Fig. 22).

Tertio, this figure shows the upper maxillary wax rim conform to this plane in a correct vertical dimension.

This concept is a procedure in order to adapt the upper maxillary to the lower mandibular maxillary.

6.5 Face-Bow

The first task should be the registration of the rotation centers and consequently, the identification of the hinge axis. After the determination of the center of rotation left and right, the face-bow is intended to translate this finding to an articulator. Unfortunately, these rotation centers are not anatomic landmarks but the geometric result of an individual and physiological components. Unfortunately, the patients are never the same and the rotation centers are not at the same level. Moreover, an intra-auricular measurement did not take into consideration the differences in the patients' auricular anatomy. Another point is that by taking maxillary landmarks as reference, the movements of the mandible guided by a neuromuscular system are ignored.

The authors came to the conclusion that face-bow transfer is not imperative to achieve better clinical results in prosthodontics, therefore, to avoid biasness in results, this system is not recommended [57] (Fig. 23).

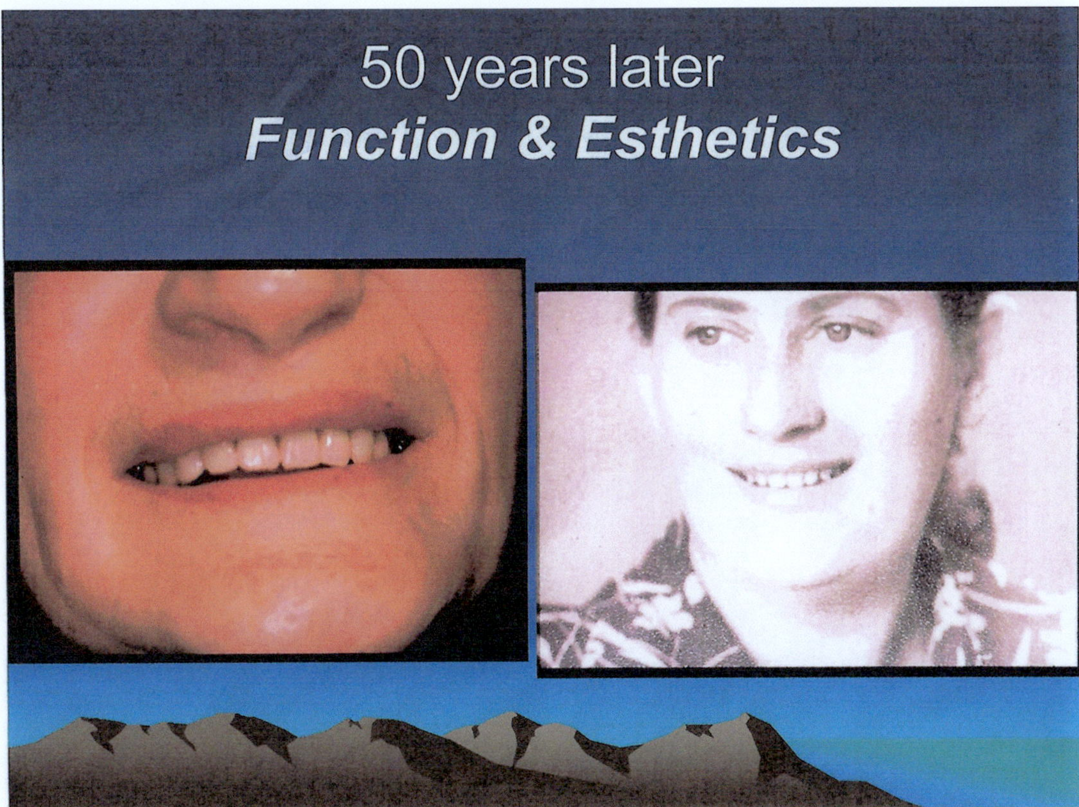

Fig. 21 Rapport tongue and occlusion

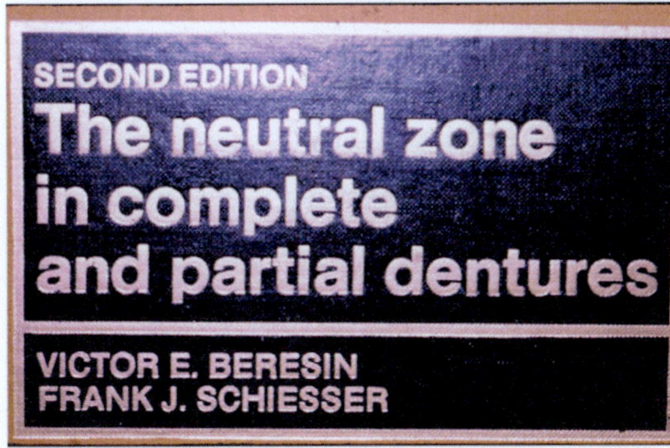

Fig. 22 Situation, tongue checks and lips

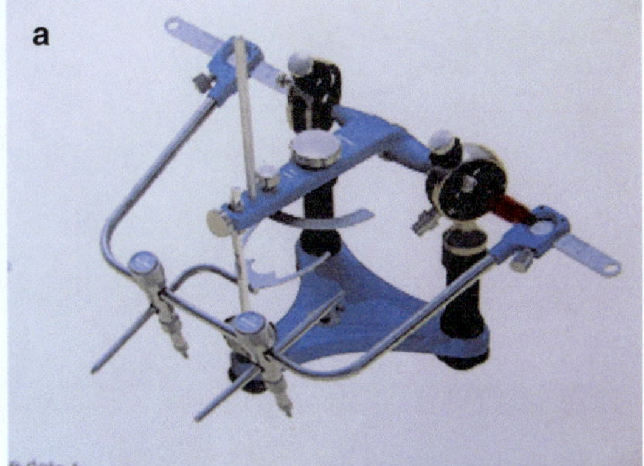

Fig. 23 (**a**, **b**) Facial asymmetry

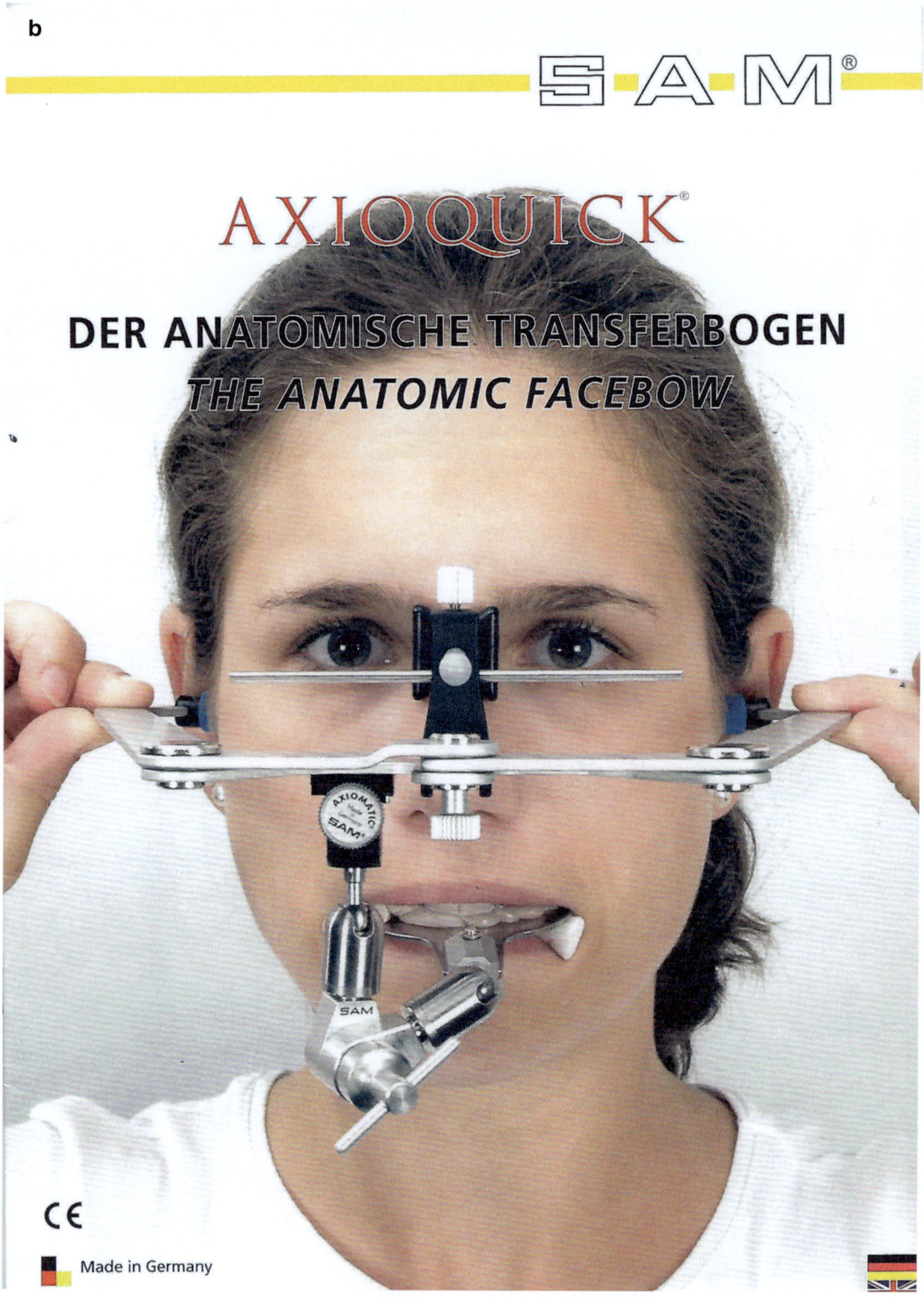

b

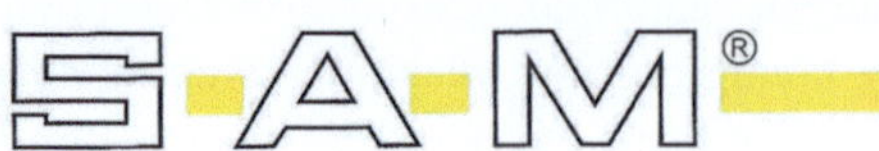

Fig. 23 (continued)

6.6 Balanced Occlusion

Since the last decades, several theories emerged, challenging a bilateral occlusal balance. In fact, this was a complex procedure since the practitioner was ignoring the occlusal landmarks: center of rotation, condylar, and anterior guidance. Nevertheless the choice of the artificial teeth was minimum of three types, i.e. anatomic, nonanatomic, and semi-anatomic. Moreover, since the mandibular movements are not symmetric, the kinetic is different from what is delivered by the articulator. Therefore, the dentist will have to handle the patient's complaints; soars, unstability and difficulty in chewing.

6.6.1 The Lingualized Occlusion

This concept allows mechanical freedom in mastication, a better food-penetration, facilitates the chairside adjustment, and minimizes the occlusal stresses [58].

The procedure is simple involving:

1. Maxillary anatomic posterior teeth with prominent lingual cusp (Fig. 24).
2. Mandible non-anatomic or semi-anatomic teeth.
3. A modification of the mandibular teeth by an elective grinding, with the collaboration of the patient performing the physiologic movement. Blatterfein, L. recommended lingualized occlusion for all removable prosthodontics. Kawai, Y. was comparing a

lingualized and fully bilateral balanced posterior occlusion for complete dentures. The result indicated a better adaptation of the dentures with a lingualized occlusion [59].

Hobo, S. demonstrates the cross point theory of the mandibular movement with the upper Maxillary teeth.

An important factor in the realization of the occlusal balance in lateral movements [60].

7 Removable Partial Denture: RPD

Numerous research studies demonstrate that one of the most important challenges in our profession is to present a prosthetic solution for senior patients. With the aging, the process of edentation involves several steps. Generally, for periodontic or systemic reasons and negligence; people lose natural teeth with time. As a result, the Edentation is frequent in the posterior segments of the mandible and the maxillae; Kennedy class 1 and 2 A premium Implant restorations are often not possible because of various barriers, mainly, anatomic obstacles, bad oral hygiene, systemic diseases, mental behavior, and economic conditions. In case of partial edentation when fixed prosthodontics is not possible, RPD remains the best choice even for a provisional restoration. But a simple acrylic device presents

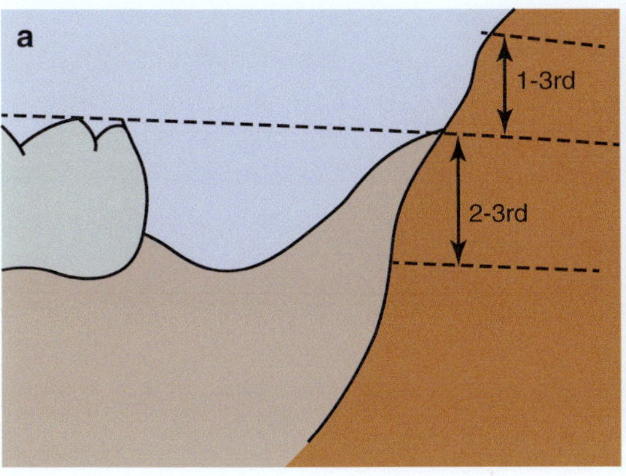

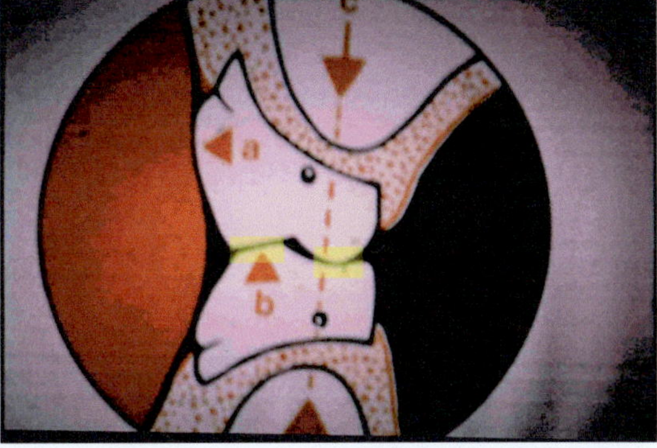

Fig. 24 (**a, b**) Lingualized balanced occlusion

obstacles regarding the hygiene, the stability, and the survival of the remaining teeth. Nevertheless, there are some major difficulties in the RPD [61].

1. <u>Poor Stability</u>
2. <u>Little Retention</u>
3. **Traumatic occlusion**
4. <u>Destruction of the Abutment by carious situation</u>
5. <u>Resorption of the supporting tissues</u>
   Strong resorption of the two or one posterior segment will, at the end, lead to a "Combination syndrome"; a collapse of the posterior vertical dimension characterized by the Flaring of the anterior teeth and the gliding of the centric forwards. In a terminal step, when the patient is edentulous, these factors are complicated to treat.
6. <u>Designing a functional RPD</u>
   To overcome this issue, and to avoid this pitfall, a metallic structure is compulsory. The design of RPD is extremely important as the realization of a Short Dental Arch (ten occluding pairs) (Fig. 25).

   Mersel, A. and his team demonstrated that utilizing the stress absorbing frame approach for partial dentures is increasing their stability and safeguarding the residual teeth [62].

   Often shortened dental arch is indicated for allowing for the tongue more space, and decreasing headaches and the temporomandibular joint pain [63] (Fig. 26).

There is also an absolute necessity to check different factors before to draft the RPD design.

The reason for instability: In Kennedy Class I or II, the distal extension is supported by the saddle, and the free end is supported by the gingiva. The difference between a fixed element and a mobile one causes a rocking movement known as the teeter-totter phenomena. In consequence, this action will drive to the loss of the most distal teeth. In order to avoid this loss, the dentist must set up an appropriate design.

(a) **Avoiding the destruction of the abutments teeth**

   An important challenge is the prevention of the supporting teeth from deterioration. For the crown-rot ratio and the Perio-dental condition, the classical recommendation is to use two twin-crowns with an indirect retainer.

(b) **Trauma absorbing by stress breakers (equalizers).**

   Retention is one of the difficult tasks. To obtain necessary retention in function (eating, speaking, and swallowing), there are two types of devices used; clasps or precisions attachments.

   More common are the clasps which are a combination of a reciprocal metallic piece and an active flexible arm. There must exists a balance between the clasp

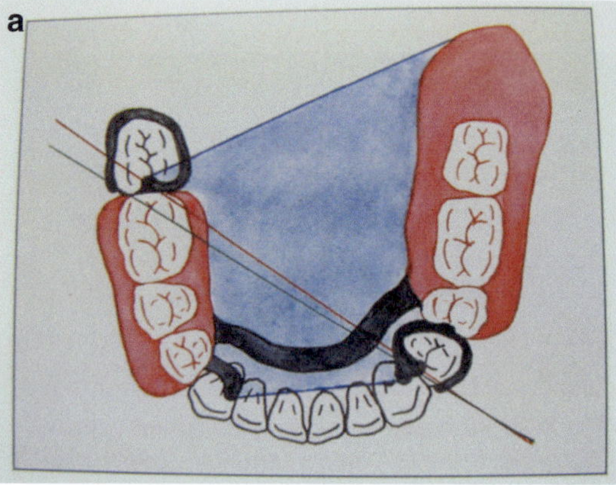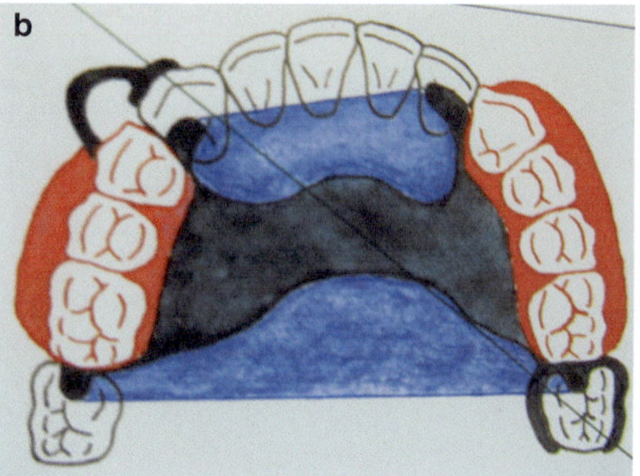

Fig. 25 (**a**, **b**) Removed partial prosthesis and function

pressure and the resistance of the teeth, which can be obtained by the localization of the rest in mesial, and with a surveyor drawing, the correct emplacement of the clasp: Mesial Rest (Fig. 27).

(c) Retainers, Stress-equalizers, Telescopes or Double-Crowns (Fig. 28).

In order to realize the preservation of the abutment teeth, stress breakers are placed to relieve the teeth from an occlusal over-loading and to keep the occlusal charge in the limits of periodontal tolerance. There are a number of prefabricated precision devices or attachments in the market;

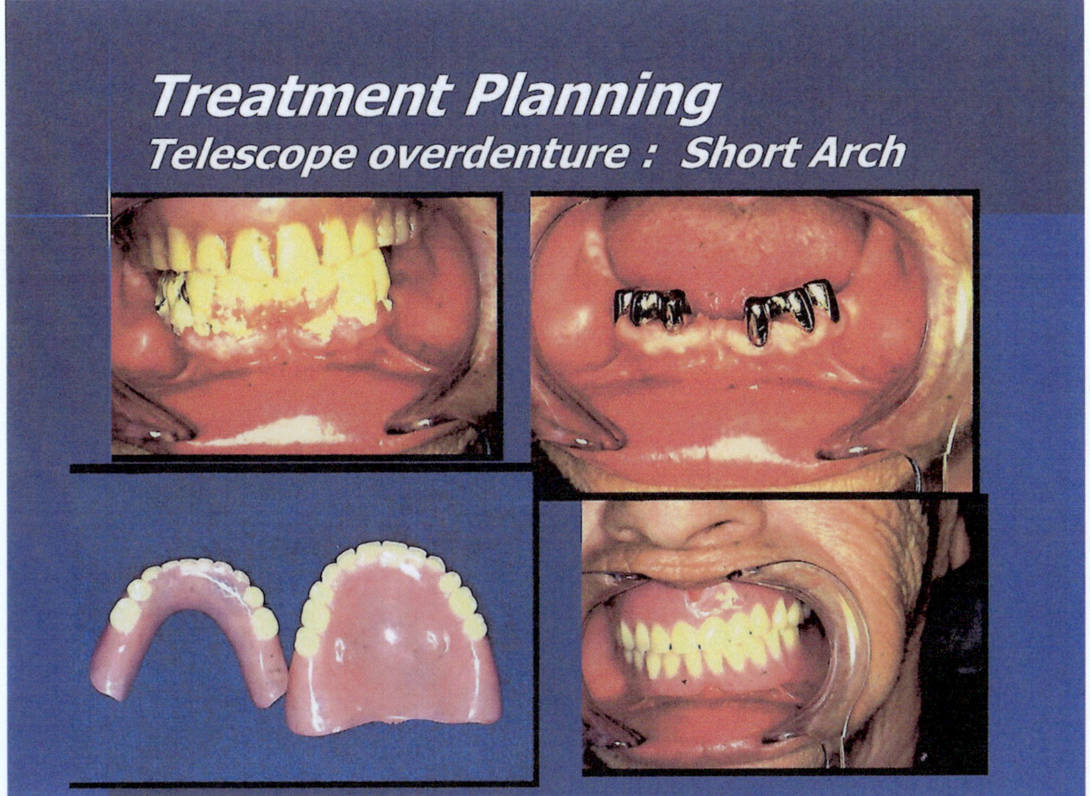

Fig. 26 Short arch denture on telescopes

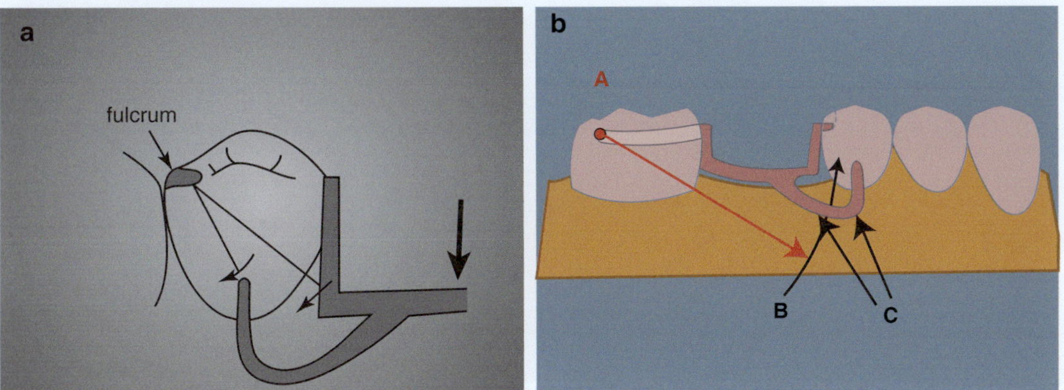

Fig. 27 (**a, b**) RPD with mesial rests

their prices are relatively high and demand a technical laboratory support. Depending on the conditions, the dentist has the choice between bars, T-Attachments, Dalbo cylindrical attachments or locators. Unfortunately, the majority of the neglected patients are in a terminal situation. The prosthetic dilemma is between the extraction of all the remaining teeth and a complete dentures restoration **or** an attempt to select some strategic teeth for necessary support of the partial dentures.

When the crown-root report does not allow a conventional crown, the oral hygiene is difficult, and when the patient has difficulties in inserting or removing his removable partial denture, the **Telescopic crown** is the best indication.

Often elders with aging have difficulties in inserting or removing their RPD [64] (Figs. 29 and 30).

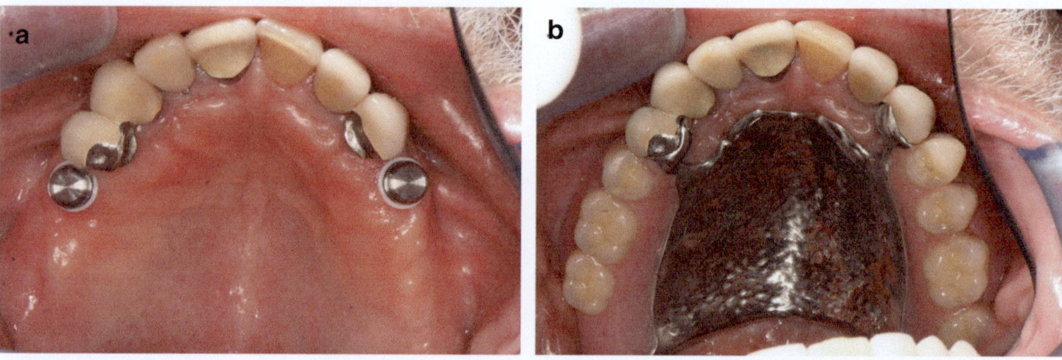

Fig. 28 (**a**, **b**) Dentures on double crown and locator

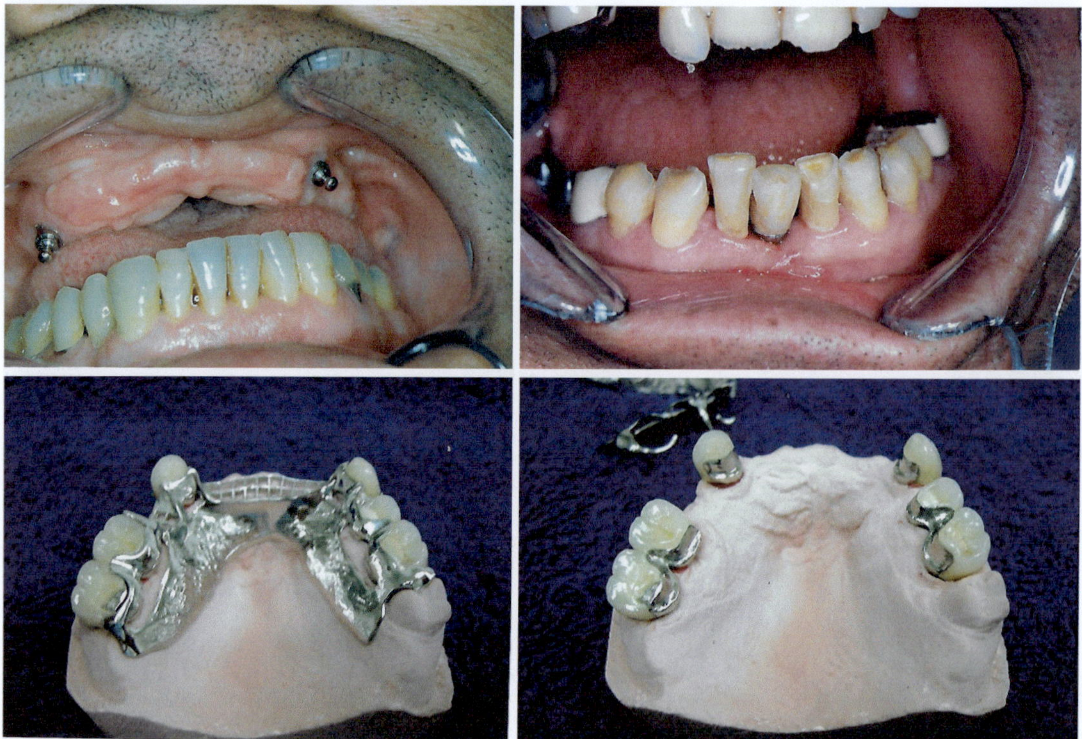

Fig. 29 RPD and crowns combination

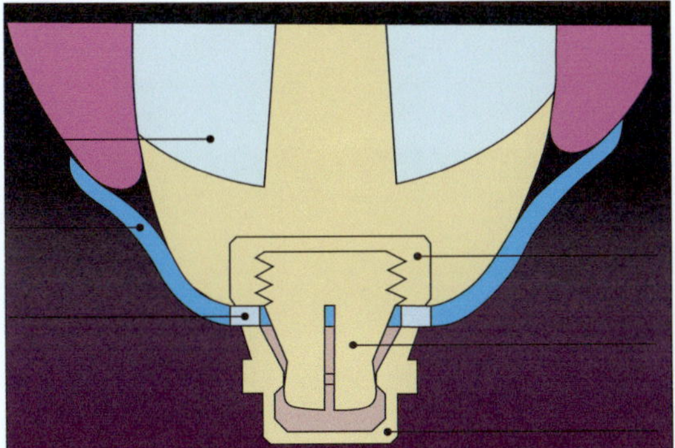

Fig. 30 CEKA attachment system

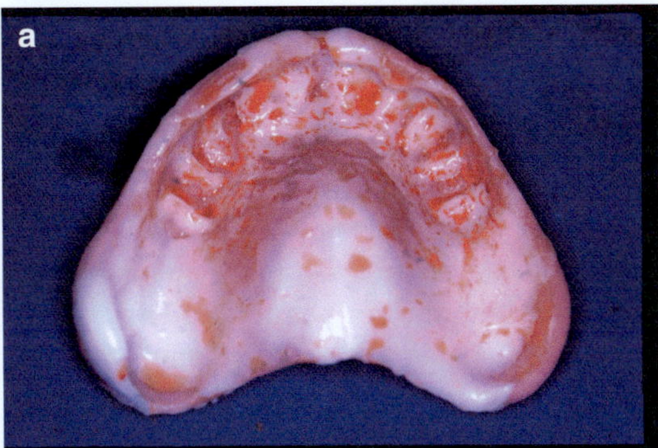

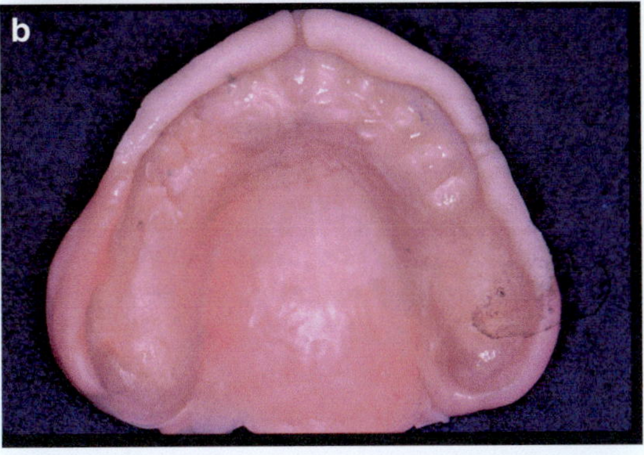

Fig. 31 (a, b) Immediate dentures soft lining insertion

Moreover, in the case of a poor prognosis, this solution can be considered a provisional or interim step. Such an minimalistic trauma will give, to the patient, an opportunity for a soft adaptation, and good hygiene.

Korb and Langer were advocating a tooth-supported telescopic prostheses in the compromised patients [65].

Other Prosthodontists as Fonseca were in favor of Maxillary or Mandibular Overlay Removable Partial Dentures for the Restoration of Worn Teeth [66].

8 Immediate or Transitional Interim Dentures

When setting up a treatment plane, the general practitioner is often skeptical about his final diagnosis. Thus, considering the complexity of all the relevant factors, before taking strategic decisions, it is wise to proceed step by step. The first principle is to give prompt help to address the acute situation without preceding to future steps, starting in this way, a true dialogue with the patient. The second step should be devoted to provide an intermediary temporary solution, creating simple prosthetic devices. The transformation of an old prosthesis is important in avoiding chair-time and high lab expenses. The third step is a period of elimination of the pathologic elements, and the estimation of the patient's adherence with the progress of his oral hygiene. This period depends on multiple factors and the evaluation is always questionable. After reaching a real stabilization, the dentist will be able to present 1–3 solutions to the patient. In this way, the final decision will be the result of a clear and kind collaboration (Fig. 31).

Beside the conventional immediate restoration of dentures, we can also note the duplicate denture procedure and an immediate denture fabrication. Because the long time of use, new dentures are the first choice. Aside the conventional immediate dentures the immediate or transitional complete dentures are presenting positive Gerodontic Considerations. The procedure is less invasive and, offers a smooth transition to the elder patient [67, 68].

In the same target a functional impression and jaw registration in a single session procedure will allow a shorter construction of the complete dentures [69].

9 Relining and Rebasing

The dentist must be aware of the difference between relining and rebasing. After surgical procedures, and serial extractions, there are important morphological changes and in this case, rebasing is necessary. Two types of rebasing are possible: the direct method, which consists of a chairside impression with the rebasing material and the indirect method, by a classical physiologic impression with polymerization in the laboratory; requiring time and finances. When the situation is not severe and the morphologic changes occurred in the prosthetic borders, to again create a perfect border molding, the dentist should utilize the same prosthetic complete denture impression technique. Attention must be paid to: the viscosity of the product, the lasting duration, and the hygiene qualities [70].

The names are different in accordance with the producer, i.e. Soft-liner, tissue-conditioner, rebasing or relining material. The dentist must explain to the patient that this procedure is only temporary, and the follow-up is compulsory. In general, this intermediary procedure facilitates the realization of the treatment plane [70] (Fig. 32).

The dentist should pay attention on the effect of resilient liner on masticatory efficiency and the general patient satisfaction in completely edentulous patients [71].

9.1 Conservative Dentistry

The Atraumatic Restorative Treatment: **ART.**

Prof. M. Goldberg highlighted the importance of the evolution of cavities to determine the effectiveness of the Glass Ionomer restorative materials. This approach will lead to a

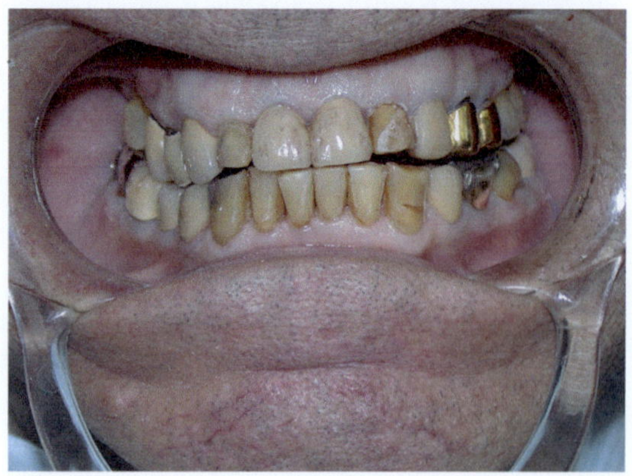

Fig. 32 Fixed prosthodontics crowns: 11, 21 after 42 year follow-up

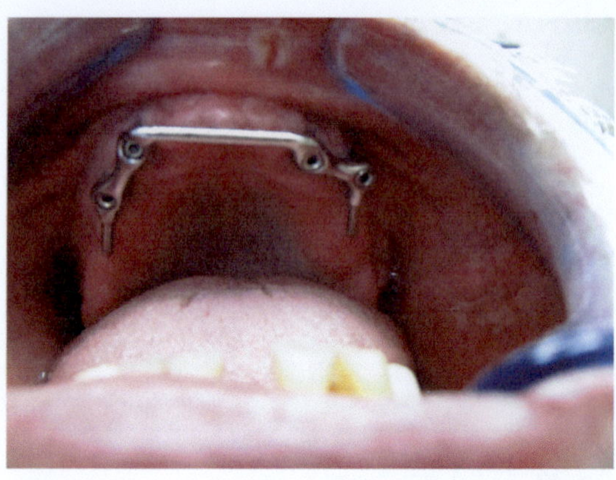

Fig. 33 Upper implant infrastructure for complete denture

Minimalistic treatment for Conservative Restorations for compromised and Elderly Patients [72].

Prof. Frencken. J.E. who introduced one of the most important concepts of MID: Minimalistic Invasive Dentistry,

He launched the Atraumatic restorative treatment utilizing high viscosity glass ionomer cement [73].

A successful experience and long-lasting results have demonstrated the universal value of this procedure in oral health (Fig. 33).

As a result of those treatments and MID approach, 75.5% of the patients stated that their oral health was better compared to the start of the treatment [74].

10 Main Obstacles for a Successful Treatment

In regard to an ethical approach, high quality treatment and satisfaction of patients are compulsory, but often with the end of the treatment, patients come back with some harsh complaints. In general, the claims are about **esthetics** and implantology.

The development of Implantology the Age – related satisfaction with Complete Dentures, the desire for improvement of the esthetics and are modifying the attitudes to an implant treatment [75] (Fig. 34).

1. During the presentation of the Treatment Plane

    The patients and their family are arguing, because of the excessive publicity, false presentation of the advantages of the new technology and unawareness of the risk factors involved. At this point, a clear and simple presentation is recommended. The practitioner must be absolutely certain that the patient has comprehensively understood his explanation.

2. After the treatment.

    If the implants fail, there is an obligation to present correct diagnostics and to look forward for a solution.

    If the restoration is not accepted, the patient can blame the dentist for restraining to refuse the implants solution.

There are three complaints that surprisingly affect the clinician:

1. **Phonetics:** The patient is able to speak, the family is able to identify his voice, but is not able to recognize the "Pronunciation." Often during mastication, there is a noise like clicking and Linguo-dental and Labio-dental sounds are affected, i.e. "S and Ch," that generate a whistling sound. A non-physiologic occlusal plane and non-adapted vertical rest dimension affect the contact with the dorsum of the tongue [76].

2. **Esthetics:**

Sometimes even the fact that the patient was happy with his dentures and felt glad to look so young, he comes back with very harsh complaints.

    "The first mistake is to show the patient his dentures" in situ "not his profile," only his face. Doing so the labial aspect appears clearly when speaking and smiling. The relation between anterior teeth and lips gives a personal touch to the restoration, if the midline is in harmony with the face? (Fig. 35).

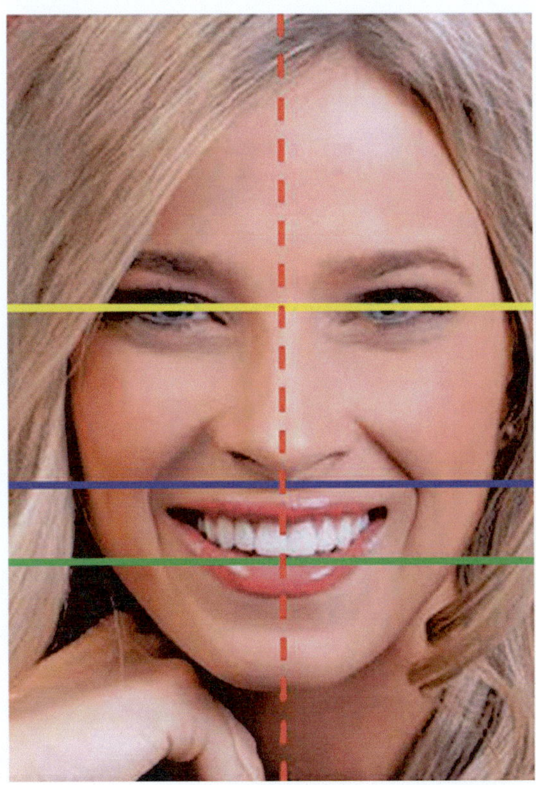

Fig. 34 Class V atraumatic restorative treatment after 9 years

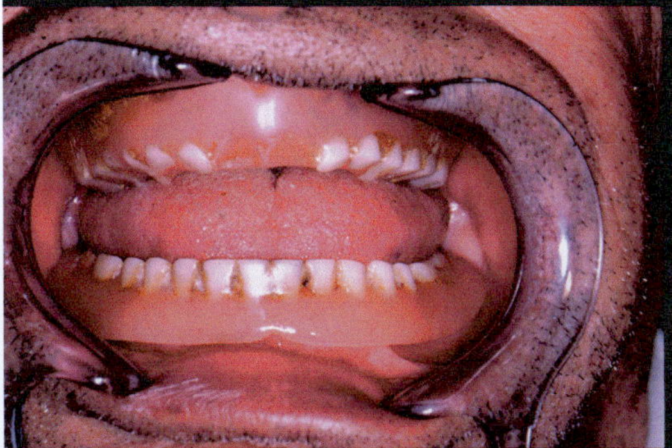

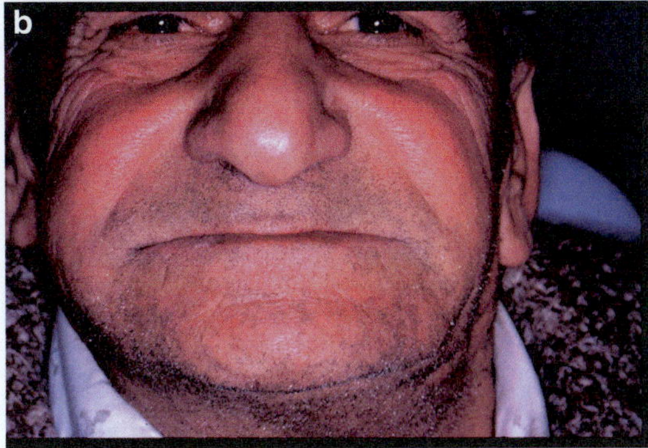

Fig. 35 (**a, b**) Vertical dimension at rest VDR and at occlusion VDO

Devi, M. and Nayar, S. were trying to determine the guidelines for Esthetics in Complete Dentures [77].

Esthetics is mainly an artistic emotion and feeling developed toward a subject. This means that every individual has his personal cultural and experience factors. By tradition, harmony is required between the different elements. In dentistry, there are basic rules giving necessary guidelines for the dentist to follow. There is an interaction between the face, the muscular and bone structures, and the teeth.

The form of the face; oval, round or square determines the form and the shape of the teeth (Fig. 36).

The color of the teeth must correspond to the shade of the skin and the eyes.

The teeth arrangement starts with the definition of the mid-line. The middle of the incisive papilla is set as the landmark of the middle. The clinician must pay attention that this point is not necessary for the middle of the face (Fig. 37).

One of the liable landmarks is the relationship between canines, incisors, and the incisive papilla [78].

Since nobody has symmetric facial structures, there could not be a similar teeth arrangement in the right and left side.

The dynamics of the lips when speaking or smiling influences the teeth arrangement and even the occlusal orientation plane in the anterior segment. Concerning the esthetics, we should focus on the color, the size, and the position of the teeth with regard to the upper and lower lip kinematics (Fig. 38).

It will be wise to involve patients during the choice. Then a real esthetic dialogue is created in order to avoid dramatic pitfalls. The best thing should be to examine old patients' photographs.

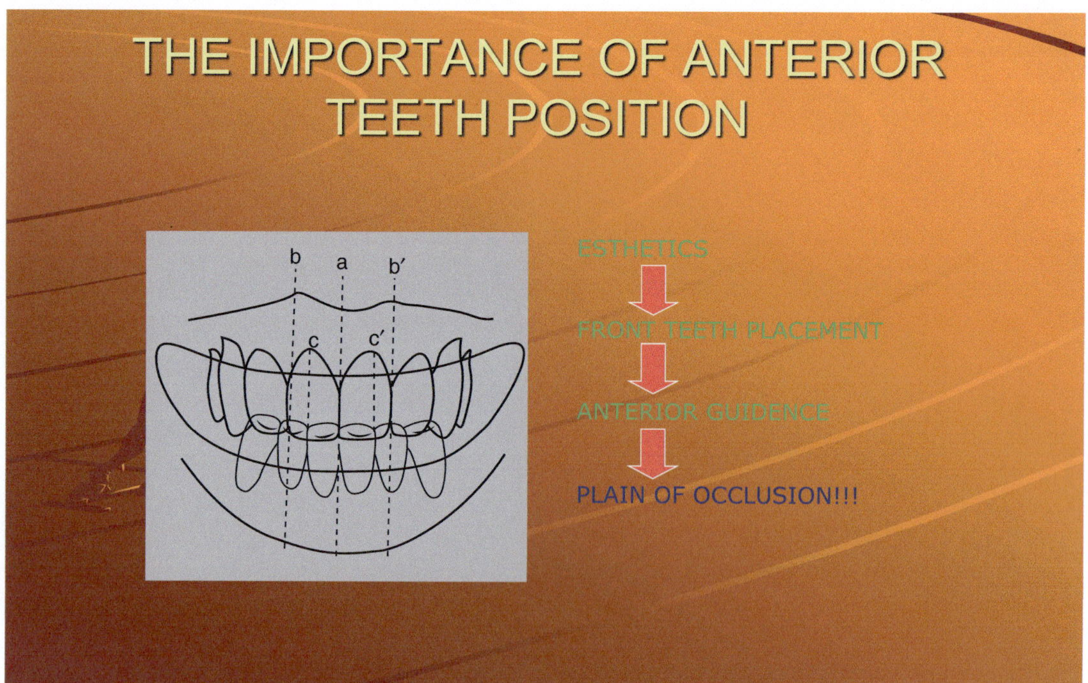

Fig. 36 Esthetic guidelines; harmony between face arch and teeth

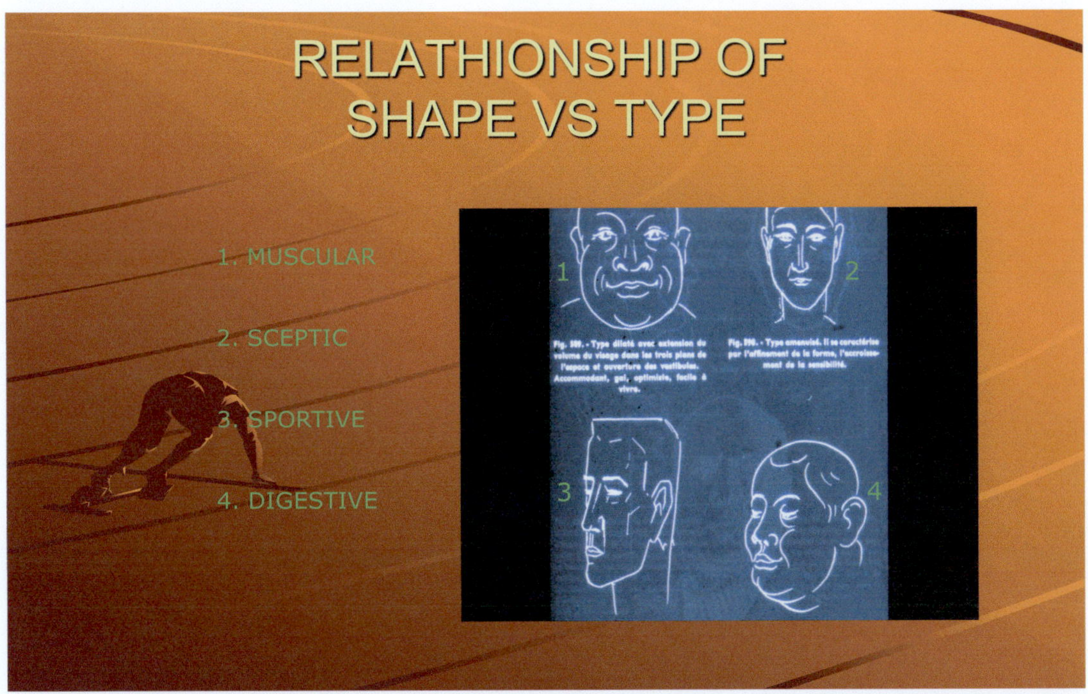

Fig. 37 Anterior teeth set up in relation with the incisive papilla

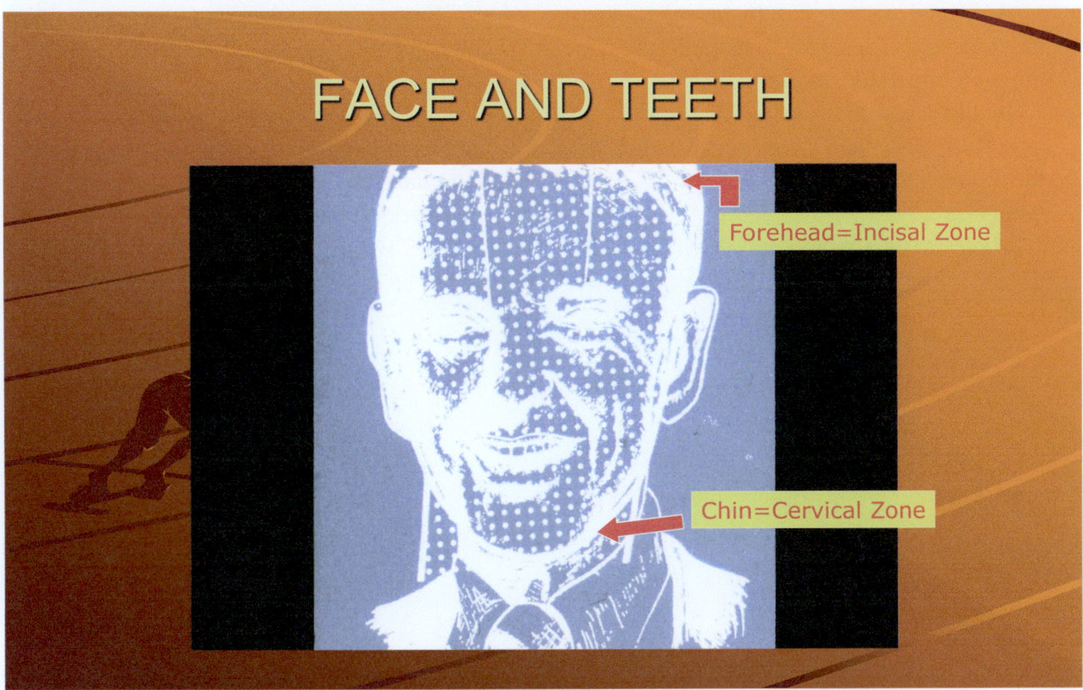

Fig. 38 Positioning the upper canines; # 13, # 23

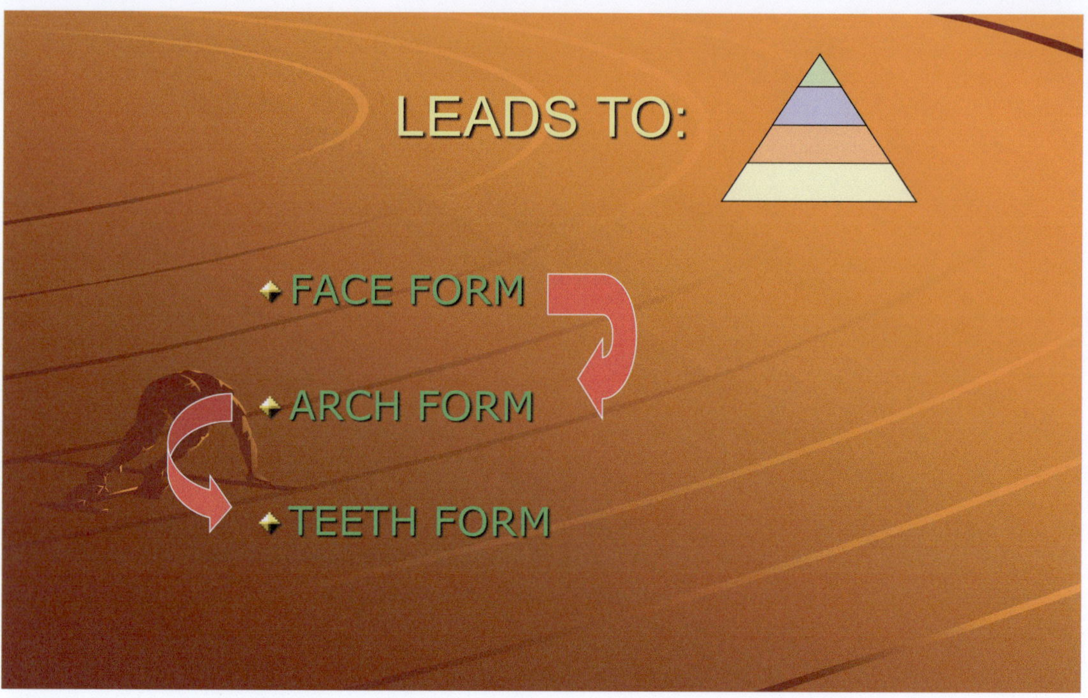

Fig. 39 Occlusal balance; working or non-working

A special session has to be schedules in order to establish a real L Esthetic dialogue, this step Imperative in Dentistry [79].

In the case of a partial restoration, the new teeth color and shape must match with the remaining teeth or partial reconstruction.

There exists a mold chart, giving the dentist the opportunity to realize an esthetic personalization of the anterior restoration (Figs. 39, 40, and 41).

3. **Occlusal Balance**

One of the most complicated factor. The dentist has to imagine the kinetic of the mastication and the position of the working and non-working teeth in the time and in the space. Obviously a Comprehensive Education should be developed (Figs. 42 and 43).

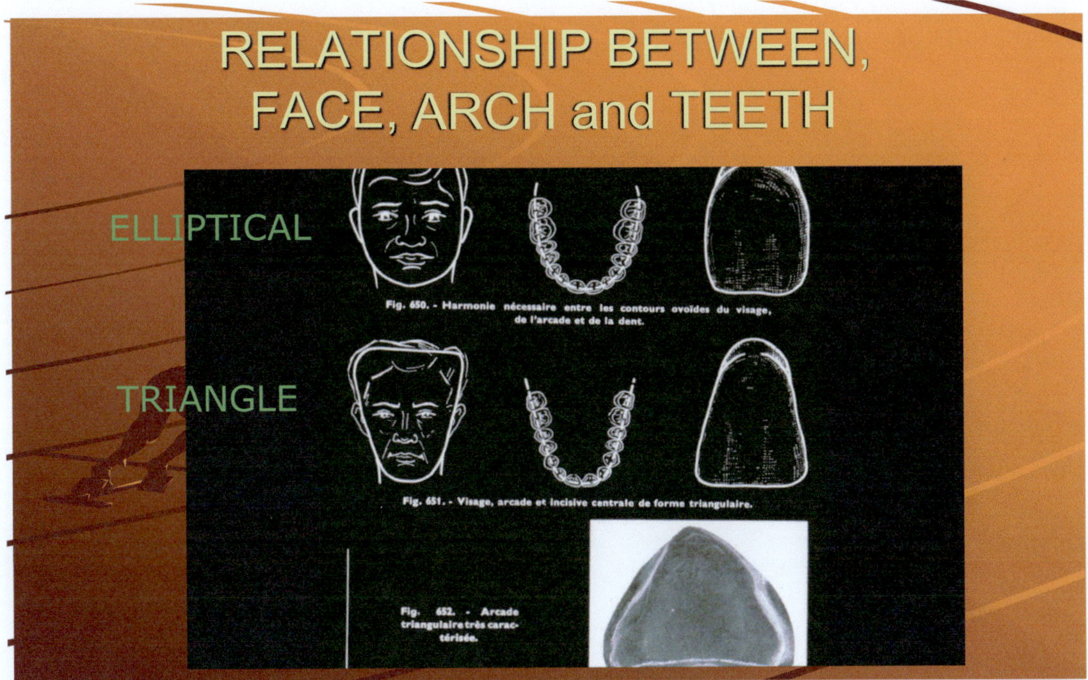

Fig. 40 A RPD support crown preparation

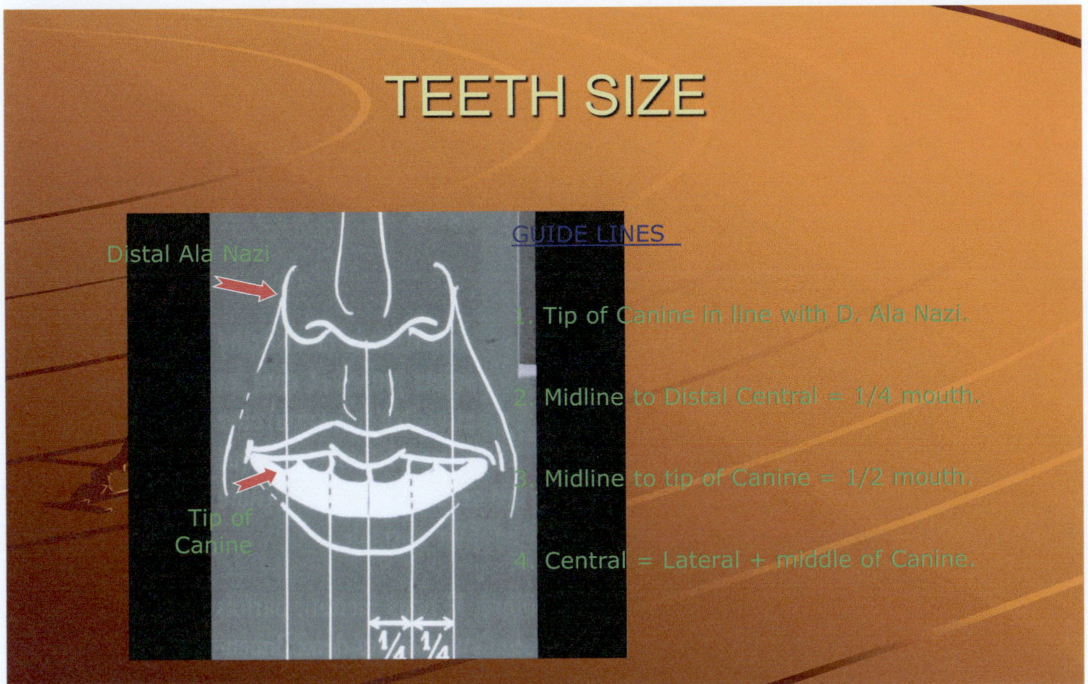

Fig. 41 Crown impression

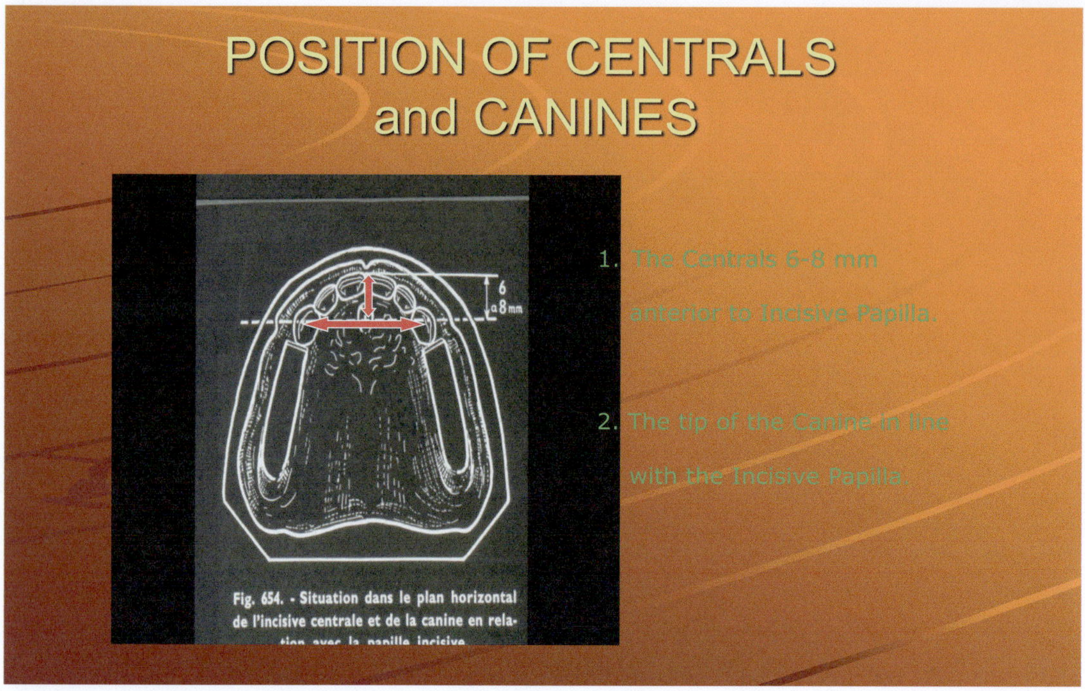

Fig. 42 Matrix technique; preparation

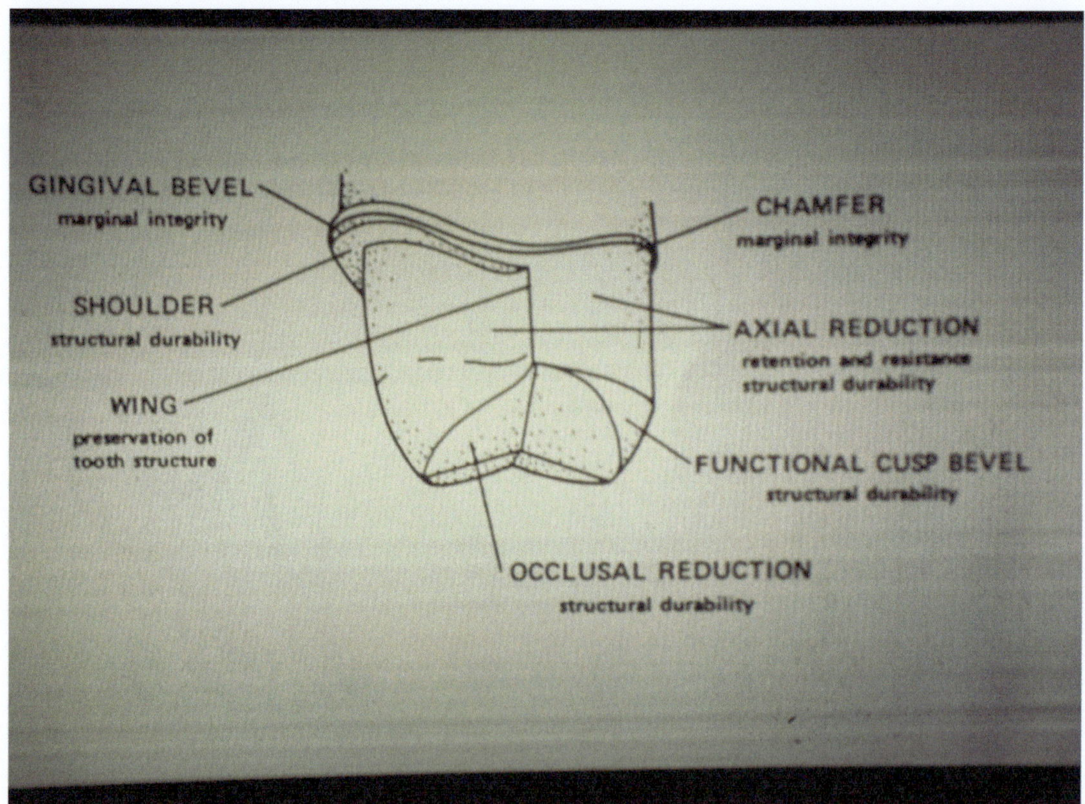

Fig. 43 Matrix final wash; Teeth preparation for a RPD supporting crown

11   Responsibility

Aside the classical barriers, often the patients come back with unexpected and embarrassing questions;

1. Why is this treatment so expensive
2. How long will your restorations be in place?
3. When should I come back for checking?

The patients are divided into several categories:

1. People who always have the feeling that your honoraria's are too expensive; on an ethical point of view, they should be explained about the specifically of treatments; including associated risks and benefits.

   In some countries, there exists a legal obligation to deliver a written financial proposal.

2. More concerned patients request to know precisely how long restorations will remain in their mouth.

   In reality, this is a difficult task, because there are numerous unknown factors as the cooperation of the patient, the global health problems and their influence on the oral health, the adherence to treatment schedule. Nevertheless, during the presentation of the treatment planning, this issue should be kindly presented and explained (Fig. 44).

3. Cooperation. Even the patient presents a cooperative attitude and develops a positive atmosphere; there is no guarantee for his behavior. The issue of the follow-up and an obligatory checking are the pretext of a habitual misunderstanding, often about esthetics (Fig. 45).

The dentist always has to remember that the patient is not a "Friend."

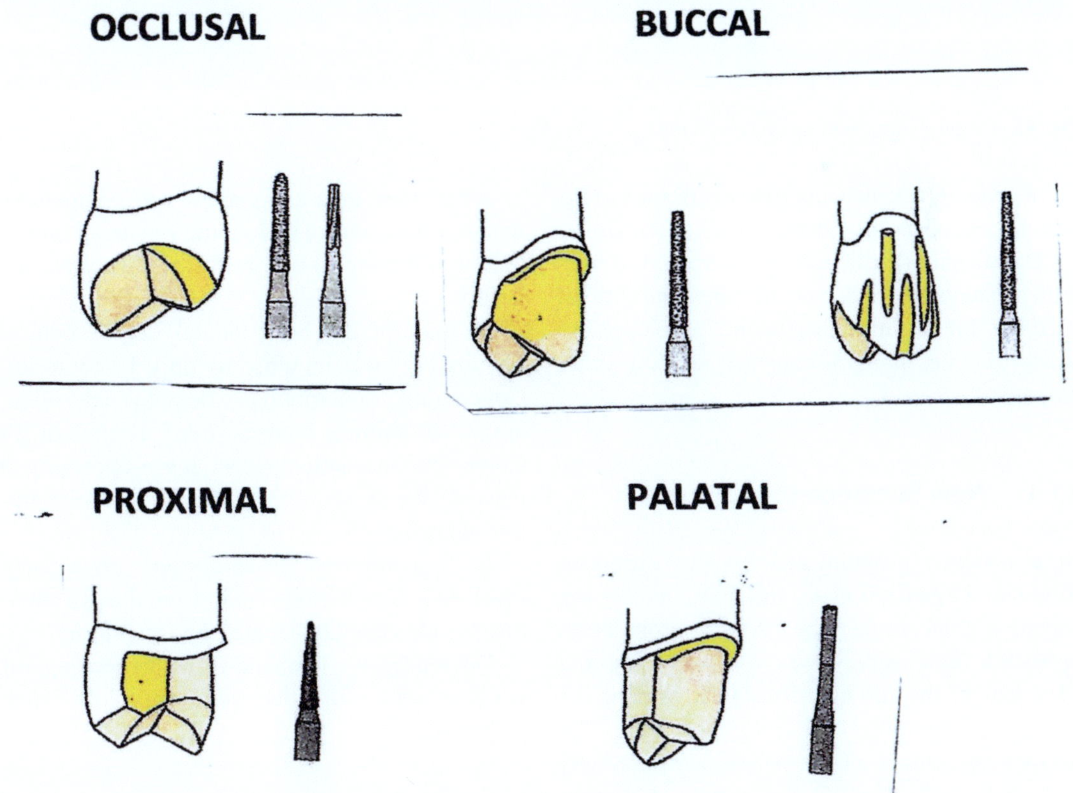

Fig. 44 Crown and RPD preparation

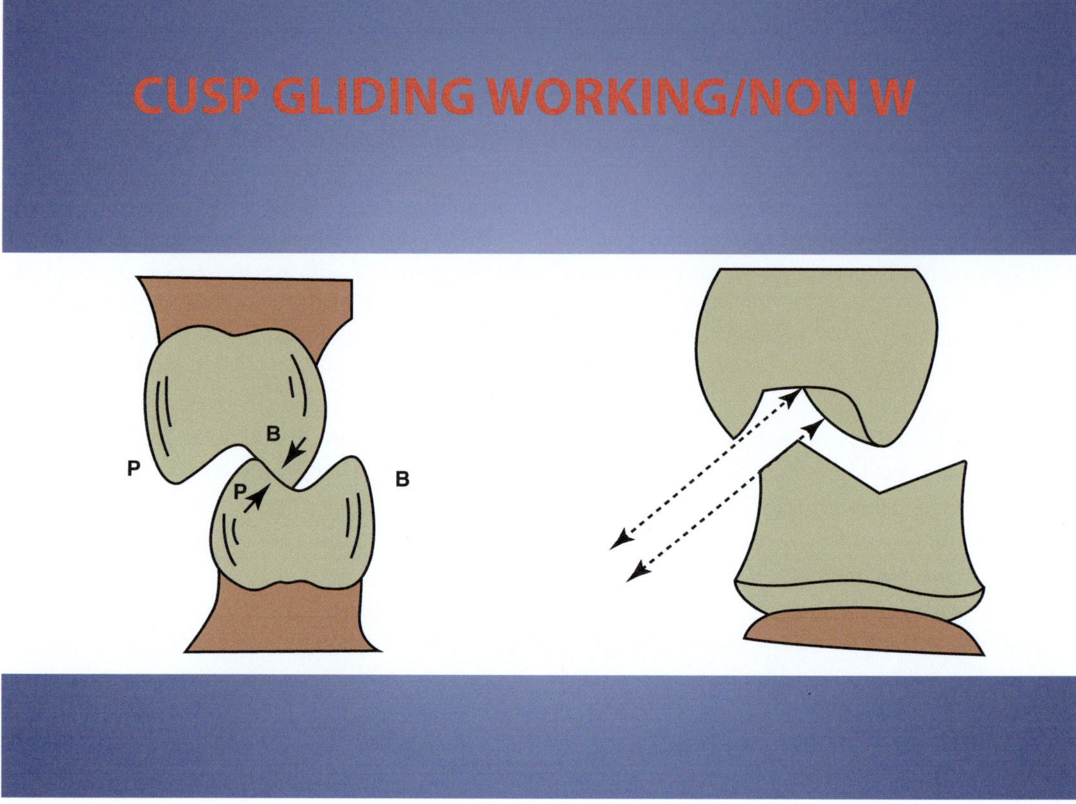

Fig. 45 Cusps gliding working / non working

In general, a dentist can treat his friends as his patients but never his patients as his friends.

The dental practitioners is committed to high ethical standards and has the responsibility of carrying out clear management, avoiding any waste of time, and consequently refusing other patients.

11.1 New Socioeconomic Impacts

In a research program led by the European Regional Organization of the FDI, interesting findings concerning the Aging Population appeared. This survey was conducted by the President of the ERO Dr Rusca Ph. Among 37 European countries, 27 (73%) took part. The average percentage of the people aged over 65 was about 20%. The life expectancy of women was higher than men 85 years vs. 80 years old.

After more than 25 years, it was compulsory to check the status of Gerodontology as an important contribution to oral health to this neglected group.

As part of the basic dental degree course, Gerontology was included by only 19 countries. Concerning continuing dental education, advanced training courses were availed in 18 Countries. On a national level, it was necessary to discover the trends of the political or administrative agenda.

In 11 countries, the authorities are actively involved in Gerodontics. Apart from this, 18 countries decided that Gerodontology is a priority.

Obviously, the financial or insurance support is necessary for the realization of such programs.

- For the nursing homes; 15 countries.
- For a nationwide support; 15 countries [80].

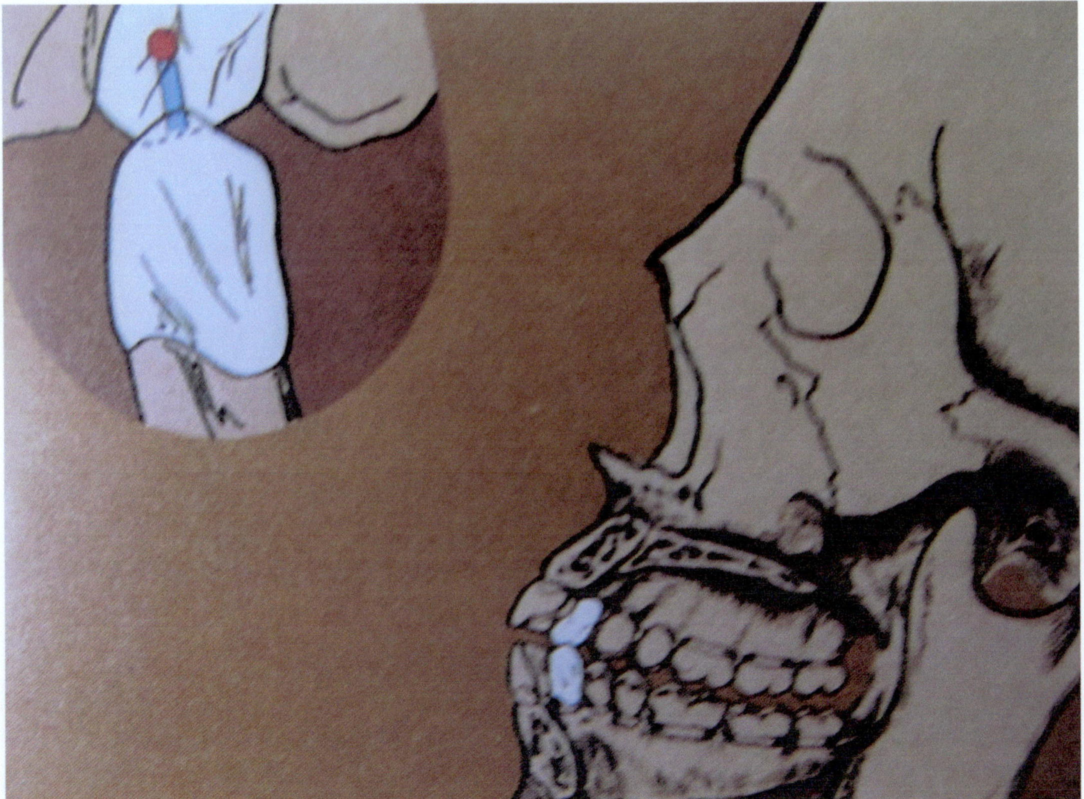

Fig. 46 Lateral movements upper and lower relationship

Another important point is the problem of the retirement age of the elderly. In the last decade, in general, the end of a professional occupation was marked at 62 years for women and 65 years for men; 34% and 28%, respectively. Since the rate of longevity is extending, the retirement age has extended to about 80 years for men and 84 for women.

Moreover, the natality is declining, so there is an important deficit in the retirement funds. People are working more years and retiring later.

As modern life has increased expenses and social security are offers less, numerous people are continuing to work mainly at home or as partial-workers. This group is consequently less flexible and restrictive about long and complicated treatment plane from the Federal Reserve Survey of Household Economics; Social Security Administration, USA (Fig. 46).

12 Fixed Prosthodontics: Crowns and Bridges

After the loss of teeth; fixed prosthetic is the ultimate solution for functional and esthetic restoration.

The actual trend is a more extensive introduction of the CAD/CAM procedure versus the old classical systems.

Concerning the target to reduce the clinical steps and financial burden for the neglected group, it is necessary to check different aspects (Fig. 47).

12.1 The Conventional Approach

The aim is to obtain a good accurate impression in one clinical step using standard products: custom or stock trays and a combination of acrylic

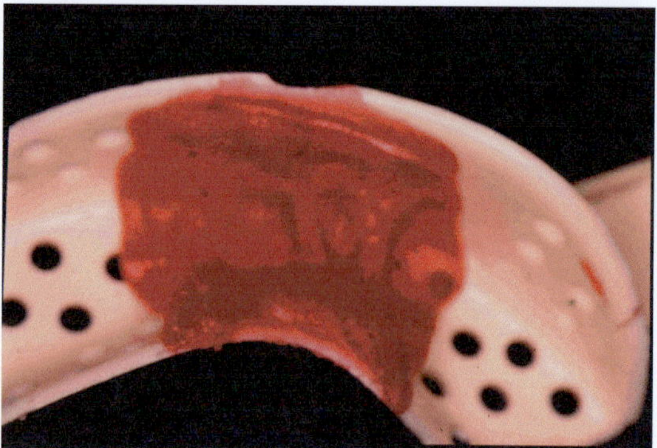

Fig. 47 Acrylic matrix for a crown impression

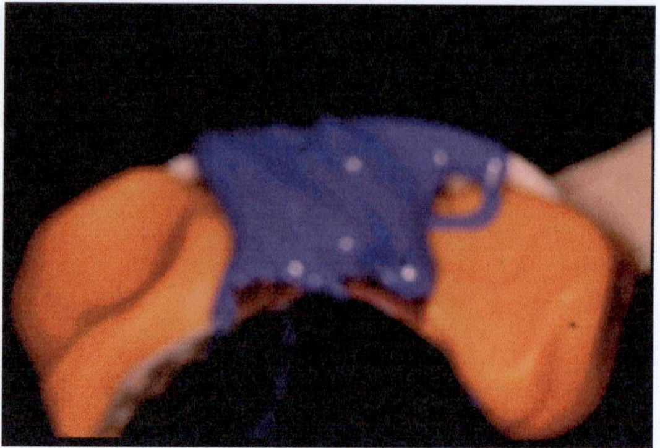

Fig. 48 Hybrid impression; puty and soft

resin and elastomer material. The result should be a perfect and readable impression. Several steps are necessary before starting the procedure.

1. A clear finishing line adapted to the anatomic and adjacent structures (Fig. 44).
2. Shaping the residual abutment preparation in the function of the teeth.
3. Checking the occlusal interaction in Centric Relation and lateral movements.

In the past, the dentists would commonly utilize the cooper tube system. The target was to utilize this concept with an acrylic self-curing formatted cooping; the *Matrix was* realized and then adjusted (Figs. 48 and 49).

Following this, a low-viscosity wash material was introduced in the matrix and quickly set in place. The matrix was not removed. In the meantime, a stock tray was filled with a putty medium elastomer. Then, the dentist would finish the impression by a classical pick-up technique (Fig. 47). The modern technologic system is in the focus these days and numerous research works are going on, but for the great majority of general practitioners working in difficult conditions, the matrix system is easier, less expensive, and overall the impression could be immediately checked.

This approach is in the right line with our attempt to reduce the treatment barrier for a great number of patients [81].

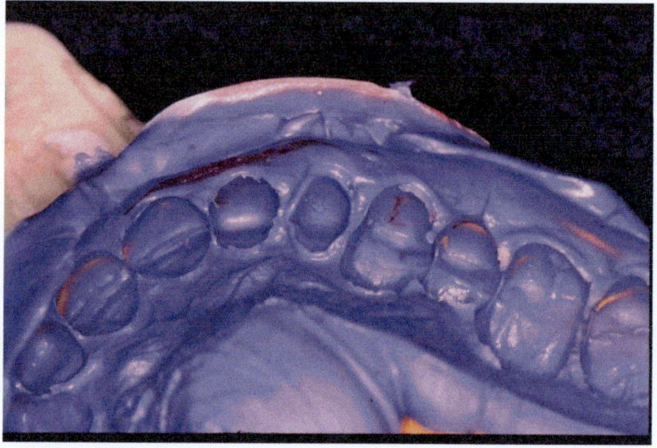

Fig. 49 Result finsl impression

The old concept of an impression with a Cooper band is now transformed in simple Crown Impression Technique, using self-curing acryl for creating a ring around the abutment tooth. Then a pick up with silicone is performed another procedure consist of as classic one step Putty –Wash Impression Technique [82].

12.2 CAD/CAM

1. Advantages include virtual setup of the design, no need for individual trays and multiple impressions, direct online contact with the laboratory, time saving, no need for metallic frame but Zirconium is used.

   It is well adapted for implant structures.
2. Limitations: The limitations include expensive material, high laboratory fees, and finan-

cial barriers for low-income population. Concerning the precision and the indications:

(a) Removable Prosthodontics; for complete denture, there is no possibility to perform a functional dynamic registration, and for the upper denture, there is no possibility of realizing vacuum retention [83].

(b) Fixed Prosthodontics; numerous researches demonstrated a marginal discrepancy as there were statistical differences between high-density polymers and the CAD/CAM system [84].

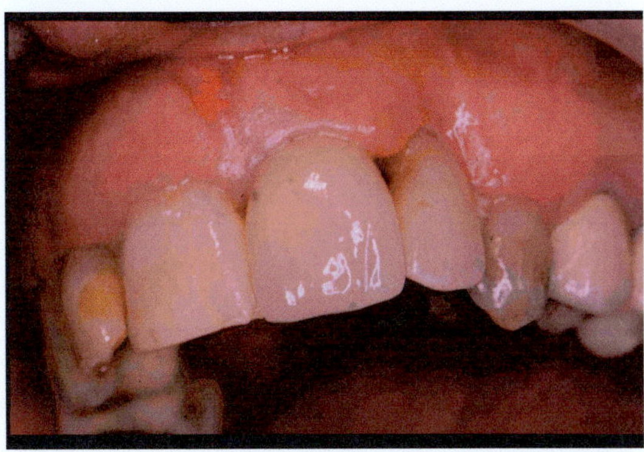

Fig. 50 Estheic and function a 10 years follow up

13 Discussion

This short memo clearly introduced a real-time situation. One has to understand the difference between morality; a universal consensus of moral obligations and ethics, the professional behavior, duties, and recommendations [85].

With the new technological trends, the practitioners are frequently exposed to difficult dilemmas. On one hand, the wishes for an oral health for all individuals are not realistic and perhaps utopic, on the other hand, for the patient waiting for a rapid, noninvasive, and cheap solution. Often the dentists are accused of over-serving or over-treatment when the medical treatment or therapy is not necessary, and in general, not appropriate. A "contrario" under-treatment is frequent by failing to treat and delaying the treatment, creating by this way, a supervised or planned inactivity.

Both attitudes are not ethical and sometimes lead to a pure "Fraud" [86] (Fig. 50).

Our modest strategy involves informing our colleagues about a range of simple procedures, time and money-saving techniques, leading to therapeutic and emotional satisfaction. Of course, people can argue that our procedure is only transitory and not complete, but ethically, it is better than to do nothing. "Primmum non Nocere" but certainly not for a long time.

As Hippocrates stated:

It is more important to know what sort of person has a disease than to know what sort of disease a person has.

Nevertheless, a new strategy appears to face the problems of the neglected patients; augmentation of the workforces by the development of new dental schools [87].

13.1 Neglected Patients vs. Ethics

It was also suggested that these schools could be ruled by private initiatives, with or without coordination of the public health authorities. In fact, such commercialization is perhaps not ethical and need a severe and strict regulation.

13.2 Dental Associations vs. Gerodontology

In a survey dealing with more than 200 dental associations, including only 55 members; 36% of them responded and unfortunately, half 18% showed some activities, specially targeting the older populations. **Oral health for an Aging Population. FDI Publication. San Francisco 2019**. Besides this, there were no basic clinical solutions presented.

We admit hereby that our publication is far to be complete and this despite the Chapters on Pedodontics, Articulations/TMJ Problems of the Prevention, and the Implants dilemma for the special patients. Therefore there IA an urgent need for as more close coordination between all the dental disciplines. In this way promoting a coherent new trend in our dental profession accordingly to the commitment to the Human Rights Declaration (WHO).

14 The COVID-19 Crisis: The Consequences in Dentistry

The epidemic of the COVID-19 is now well known. The symptomatic is daily explained to the population: Fever, head ache, cold, cough, asphyxiation, agenesy, anosmia (Loss of taste and loss of smell). Sometimes oral vesiculobullous lesions and periodontal pathologies [88].

The Pattern of Transmission is very basic and simple. The interpersonal transmission is via respiratory droplets and close contacts. The nose and the mouth are the major gateways.

The dramatic implementation is a permanent proximity (in average t5–20 cm) of the dentist and the COVID-19. Consequently, major changes should be introduced in the management of our profession.

Since this pandemic concerns all the population; the problems are not only devoted to the Profession but also to the Public Health Consequences: The total population should be considered as a Vulnerable Group.

The economic burden and the socio-economic imperatives will greatly influence the Patients ability of the pay their treatments. Saying this signify that the treatment strategies must be focused for a comprehensive adapted approach, as descripted briefly in our book.

15 Conclusion

To summarize, our main targets are to bring a solution to the questions; what amount of suffering and damage is acceptable in Our Society. Is our Profession actually aware for conceptual change and ready binging our contribution to happy end? Therefore, there is a need for close coordination between all the dental disciplines to promote a coherent new trend in our profession according to the commitment to the ethical principles by the FDI declaration. This book is not a classical textbook even not a manual but more a manifestation and also a signal for a better Global Oral Health. We hope now that this manuscript will bring some practical and clinical achievements. We are waiting to hear comments and remarks; an important element for a common interesting road map.

References

1. Newton JT, et al. Changing patient oral health behavior. Br Dent J. 2017;23:147–50.
2. Mersel A, Peretz B. A behavioral approach in the treatment of elderly patients: a new philosophy. Int Dent J. 2003;53(1):51–6.
3. Dartevelle S, Fukai K. An in depth looks at oral health in aging. FDI.org/news. 20180711. 2008.
4. Mersel A. An adapted continuing education program in Gerodontics: the actual challenge. J Glob Oral Health. 2019;1:1–5. https://doi.org/10.25259/JGOH-6-2019.
5. Kossioni A, et al. An expert opinion from the European College of Gerodontology and the European Geriatric Medicine Society: European Policy Recommendations on Oral Health for Older adults. J Am Geriatr Soc. 2018;66(3):609–13.
6. Visschere L, et al. Dentist's opinion in Belgium on the barriers providing oral care to frail older people. Clin Oral Investig. 2015; https://doi.org/10.1007/s00784-015-1652.
7. Foltyn P. Ethical decision making in aged care. Gerodontology. 2017;34:289–90.
8. Berkey D, et al. The old-old patient the challenge of clinical decision making. J Am Dent Assoc. 1996;127:321–31.
9. Ettinger R, et al. Curriculum content in geriatric dentistry in USA dental schools. Gerodontology. 2017;35(1):1–4.
10. Calache MS, et al. Minimum intervention dentistry – a new horizon in public dental care. Aust Dent J. 2013;58(1):17–25.
11. Muller F, et al. What are the prevalence and incidence of tooth loss in adult and elderly population in Europe. Clin Oral Implants Res. 2007;18(3):2–14.
12. Calleja-Sordo E, et al. Novel Ethical dilemmas arising in geriatric clinical practice. Med Health Care Philos. 2014; https://doi.org/10.1007/s11019-014-9593-6.
13. MacEntee MI. Clinical Epidemiology concerns and the geriatric prosthodontic patient. J Prosthet Dent. 1994;72:487–91.
14. Mersel A, et al. The Time factor: one of the major elements in the therapeutic evaluation in Gerodontology. J Glob Oral Health. 2018;1(1):1–4.
15. Farooq A. Dental anxiety. Understanding this key to an effective management. Dent Update. 2016;43:883–90.

16. Mersel A, Lowenthal U. Anxious anticipation of complete dentures. Spec Dent. 1996;5–6:29–31.
17. Soeli MH, et al. The oral cavity of elderly patients in diabetes. Diabetes Metab. 2007;33(1):1–18.
18. Avivi-Arber L, Sessie BJ. Jaw sensomotor control in healthy adults and defects of aging. J Oral Rehabil. 2017;45:1–25. https://doi.org/10.1111/jour.12554.
19. Hassona Y, et al. Oral cancer early detection –a pressing needs for continuing education in Jordan. Asian Pac J Cancer Prev. 2015;16–17:7727–30.
20. Zengarini E, et al. Fatigue. Relevance and implications in the aging population. Exp Gerontol. 2015;70:1–27.
21. Coelho LS. Medication in elderly people: it's influence on salivary patterns, signs and symptoms of dry mouth. Gerodontology. 2010;27:129. https://doi.org/10.1111/j.1741-2358.00293x.2009.
22. Guarnzo-Herreno CC, et al. Oral Health and welfare state regimes: a cross national analysis of European countries. Eur J Oral Sci. 2013;121:168–75.
23. Sheiham A. Oral health, general health and quality of life. Bull World Health Organ. 2005;83(9):644.
24. Schipper L. et al. 2014. https://doi.org/10.1016/j.Health.OP.07020.
25. Alotaibli MT, et al. Are there rural-urban differences in dentists supply? EC Dent Sci. 2019;18(8):1784–90.
26. Ogunbodede EO. Population ageing and the implications for Oral Health in Africa. Gerodontology. 2013;30:1–2.
27. Marchini L, et al. Geriatric dentistry education and context in a selection of countries in 5 continents. Spec Care Dent. 2018;38:123. https://doi.org/10.1111/scd.12281.
28. Kossioni A, et al. Higher education in gerodontology in European universities. BMC Oral Health. 2017;17:71. https://doi.org/10.1186/s12903-017-0362-9.
29. Nitschke I, et al. Under graduate teaching in gerodontology. Gerodontology. 2004;21:23–129.
30. Yamalik N, Mersel A, et al. Analysis of the extent and efficiency of the partnership and collaboration between the Dental Faculties and the National Dental Associations within the FDI-ERO zone. A dental faculty 's perspective. Int Dent J. 2015;12045:1–4.
31. Yamalik N, Mersel A, et al. Collaboration between Dental Faculties and National Dental Associations within the FDI–ERO a NDS perspective. Int Dent J. 2011;1(61):307–13.
32. Yao CS, Mac Entee MI. Inequity in oral health care for elderly Canadians. Part 2. Causes and ethical considerations. J Can Dent Assoc. 2014;80:10–8.
33. Suomalainen K, et al. Guidelines for the organization of continuing professional development activities for the European Dentist. Eur J Dent Educ. 2013;17(1):29–37.
34. Council of European Dentists. Code of ethics for the dentist in the European Union. Eurodental. 2017:3–6.
35. Mersel A, et al. The difficulties of the continuing education in geriatric dentistry: analysis. Indian J Dent Res. 2018;29(5):541–3.
36. Mersel A, et al. Evaluation in continuing education. Dent Asia. 2013;7–8:1–4.
37. Mersel A. Speaker guidelines lecturing in continuing education. Dent Asia. 2013;9–10:5–53.
38. de Vries N, et al. Ethical dilemmas in elderly patients. A perspective from the ethics of care. Clin Geriatr Med. 2012;28:93–104.
39. Carlsson G. Critical review of some dogmas in Prosthodontics. J Prosthodont Res. 2008;53:3–10.
40. Frias-Neto A. Bilateral articulation: science or dogma. Dent Update. 2014;41:428–30.
41. Marchini L. Patient's satisfaction with complete dentures an update. Spec Care Dent. 2014;17(4):5–8.
42. Beresin V, Shiesser F. The neutral zone in complete dentures. 2nd ed. St Louis, MO: C. V. Mosby; 1978.
43. Klein A. Piezographic prosthodontics. In: Libbey J, editor. Prothese piezograhique; 1988. ISBN 0-86196-141-2.
44. Mersel A. A contemporary prosthetic challenge. Part-1: Mandibular impression technique. Gerodontology. 1987;6(1):79–81.
45. Mersel A, Eisenberg G. Physiological design of the complete dentures space. Dent Asia. 2012;11–12:24–6.
46. Srinivasan M, et al. CAD/CAM milled removable complete dentures: an in vitro evaluation of trueness. Clin Oral Investig. 2017;21:2007. https://doi.org/10.1007/s00784-016-1989-7.
47. Goodacre CJ, et al. CAD/CAM fabricated complete denture concepts and clinical methods of obtaining required morphological data. J Prosthet Dent. 2012;1:1–10.
48. Meaney S, et al. Qualitative investigations into patient's perspectives on edentulouness. Gerodontology. 2015;4:79–85.
49. Tau S, Mersel A. Spatial relationship between anatomic landmarks in edentulous patients: a radiographic study. J Prosthet Dent. 1983;50(3):314–8.
50. Murat E, et al. Radiographic evaluation of alveolar ridge heights of dentate and edentulous patients. Gerodontology. 2012;29:7–23.
51. Sears VH. Principles and technics for complete dentures constructions. St Louis, MO: C. V. Mosby; 1949.
52. Mersel A. Atypical edentulous patients: a gerodontic approach. Dent Asia. 2007;3–4:31–4.
53. Bhupinder K, et al. Tongue: the most disturbing element in mandibular denture. How to handle it? Ann Dent Res. 2012;2(1):44–51.
54. Bohnenkamp DM, Lily T. Phonetic and tongue position to improve mandibular denture retention: a clinical report. J Prosthet Dent. 2007;98:414–347.
55. Chalapathi R. Inclined plane effect and leverage perspectives of stable dentures. Ann Prosthodont Restorat Dent. 2016;7–9(2–3):63–8.
56. Nisizaki S, Nokubi T. Manual of piezography. Reproduction of the prosthodontic space. Osaka: Japan SIPAF; 1999. p. 1–23.
57. Gyun D, et al. Reliability of an ear-face bow transfer instrument. J Prosthet Dent. 1999;82(2):150–5.
58. Blatterfein L, et al. Lingualized occlusion for removable prosthodontics. J Prosthet Dent. 2025;38(6):599–718.

59. Kawai Y. Clinical trial comparing lingualized and fully bilateral balanced posterior occlusion for complete dentures. J Prosthet Res. 2017;61:113. https://doi.org/10.1016/j.2016.
60. Hobo S. Cross point theory of the mandibular movement. Quintessence Int. 1993;10(250):1051–63.
61. McKenna G, et al. The impact of rehabilitation using removable partial dentures and functionally oriented treatment on oral health-related quality of life. A randomized controlled clinical. J Dent. 2015;43:66–71.
62. Mersel A. Stress absorbing frame approach for partial edentate patients. Dent Asia. 2008;5–6:34–9.
63. Riesman DR, et al. Effect of shortened dental arch on Temporo-Mandibulat Joint intra-auricular disorders. J Oral Facial Pain Headache. 2018;32–3:329–37.
64. Hamalainen P, et al. Oral Health status change in handgrip strength over a 5 years period in 80 year old people. Gerodontology. 2004;21:5–160.
65. Langer A, Langer Y. A tooth supported telescopic protheses in compromised conditions: a clinical report. J Prosthet Dent. 2000;84(2):129–31.
66. Fonseca J, et al. Maxillary overlay removable partial dentures for the restoration of worn teeth. Inside Dent Technol. 2012;12(1):2–9.
67. Caputi S. Immediate denture fabrication: a clinical report. Ann Stomatol. 2013;3–4:273–7.
68. Mersel A, et al. Immediate or transitional complete dentures: gerodontic considerations. Int Dent J. 2002;52–4:298–303.
69. Utz KH, et al. Functional impression and jaw registration a single session procedure for the construction of complete dentures. J Oral Rehabil. 2001;31:554–61.
70. Mersel A. Immediate dentures: rebasing or relining dental Asia. Adv Board Quot. 2012;5–6.
71. Mangtani N, et al. Effect of resilient liner on masticatory efficiency and general satisfaction in completely de nulous patients. Dent Spcial. 2015;3(2):10–155.
72. Goldberg M. Minimalistic approach for conservative restorations: oral restorations or compromised and elderly patients. Cham: Springer Nature; 2019. p. 121–40. Chapter 8.
73. Frenken JE. Atraumatic restorative treatment and minimal Intervention in Dentistry. Br Dent J. 2017;223:183–9.
74. Da Mata C, et al. Subjective impact of MID in Oral Health of elder's patients. Clin Oral Investig. 2014;16:681. https://doi.org/10.1007/84-014-1290-6.
75. Mueller F, et al. Age related satisfaction with complete dentures, desire for improvement and attitudes to implant-treatment. Gerodontology. 1994;11(1):7–12.
76. Jain CD, et al. Phonetics in dentistry. Int J Dent Med Res. 2014;1(1):31–7.
77. Devi KH, Nayar S. Esthetics in complete dentures. J Dent Med Sci. 2018;17(7):41–5.
78. Mersel A, Ehrich J. Relationship between canines, incisors and the Incisive Papilla. Quintessence Int. 1981;12(9):1–3.
79. Mersel A. Le dialogue esthetique. Imperatif en Dentisterie Geriatrique Questions d'Odontologie. 1982;26:389–91.
80. Rusca P. Ageing population. 2019. www.erodental.org/organs-and-bodies/plenary-session-San-Francisco-Minutes.
81. Livatditis GJ. Comparison of the new Matrix system with traditional fixed prosthodontic impression procedures. J Prosthet Dent. 1998;79(2):200–7.
82. Mersel A, Eisenberg G. A simple crown impression technique. Dent Asia J. 2008;5–6:34–9.
83. Chebib N, et al. Edentulous Jaw impression techniques: a vivo comparison of trueness. J Prosthet Dent. 2019;121:1–8. https://doi.org/10.1016/j.prosdent.2018.08.016.
84. Yilmaz B, et al. Marginal discrepancy of CAD—CAM complete arch supported frame works. J Prosthet Dent. 2018;120–1:65–70.
85. Golder S, et al. Attitudes toward the ethics of research using social media: a systematic review. J Med Internet Res. 2017;19(6):1–24.
86. Sykes LM, et al. In my mouth Part 1: Ethical concerns regarding dental over-treatment and under-treatment. S A Dent J. 2017;12(8):281–3.
87. Mersel A, Mann J, Vered Y. A new approach in continuing education. Dent AsiaDent Manag. 2012;3–4:30–3.
88. Badran ZX, et al. Oral vesiculobullous lesions and perio-dental pathologies. Elsevier Medical Hypotheses. Amsterdam: Elsevier; 2020. p. 140–09.

Prevention for Vulnerable Patients: Atraumatic Carious Treatment and Mild-to-Moderate Periodontal Therapy

Michel Goldberg

1   Introduction

For years pediatric dentistry and adult therapies involving dental cares have used and prepared according to Black's classification [1]. This operative and restorative dentistry implicates that the preparation of cavities removed also sound tissues. The shape of the cavities were aiming to prevent recurring lesions and also were prepared according to geometrical and mechanical reasons. The different classes of cavities were planned in order to be filled by biomaterials deprived of adhesive properties such as gold aurifications, inlays/onlays, silver amalgam, and phosphate-containing cements. All these sophisticated preparations imply an adaptation to mechanical commitments. With the evolution of the properties of recent biomaterials, the concepts have evolve taking in consideration the adhesive properties of biomaterials that have modified the classical concepts, according to the recent knowledge on the carious diseases. It is also clear that periodontal inflammation (gingivitis) may give rise to a more severe periodontal disease (periodontitis). Prevention of periodontal diseases may contribute to reduce clinical procedures implying expensive periodontal therapies, namely for vulnerable patients, or underdeveloped countries.

Vulnerable patients include elderly cohorts, handicapped individuals needing special care treatments, and undeserved children's. These patients should be the beneficiary of prevention. The questions to be solved are: how to maintain a healthy aging population, how to treat handicapped children's and to adults which are needing special cares, and how to manage the social and economic needs (Mersel; chapter in press).

Prevention of the carious and periodontal diseases is oriented toward four distinct treatment designs:

- **Primary prevention:** It focuses on preventing new cases of oral diseases. It uses collective prevention measures such as fluoridation of water and/or school oral health programs. At the individual size, primary prevention aims to prevent the early colonization of children's teeth by cariogenic bacteria. Prevention also includes the management of other factors, avoiding cariogenic diet rich in fermentable carbohydrates, aggravated by poor oral hygiene habits.
- **Secondary prevention:** It is oriented on the prevention of the disease already established and progressing. This includes screening the patients to detect carious lesions and gingival

M. Goldberg (✉)
Department of Oral Biology, Faculty of Fundamental and Biomedical Sciences, INSERM UMP-S1124, Paris Cité University—Biomedicale des Saint Pères, Paris, France

© The Author(s), under exclusive license to Springer Nature Switzerland AG 2022
A. Mersel (ed.), *Treatment Dilemmas for Vulnerable Patients in Oral Health*,
https://doi.org/10.1007/978-3-031-08435-5_2

inflammation at the earliest possible stage so that appropriate treatment can be delivered.

- **Tertiary prevention:** It aims to prevent recurrence of the diseases as well as the failure of preventive and restorative care initially implemented.
- **Quaternary prevention:** It aims to identify at risk of overmedicalization, to protect the patients from new medical invasion and suggest interventions which are ethically acceptable. It avoids the consequences of unnecessary or excessive intervention of the health system. Actions that prevent iatrogenesis and disease mongering refer to the advertisements of drug (pharmaceutical) companies and insurers, implying overmedicalization, drugs misuse, in order to expand the markets for treatments.

With regard to the evolution of treatment, ART, pioneered in the mid-1980s in Tanzania, is based on the removal of soft carious dentin using hand instruments alone, keeping intact the partially demineralized affected dentin, and restoring the cavity with an adhesive material, namely the glass-ionomer cements (GIC) [2]. The evolution of the shape of cavities avoid nowadays drilling, the preparation of undercuts, for the treatment of caries. For the periodontal tissues, how to stay at a stage of a reversible gingivitis rather to move toward a non-reversible chronic periodontitis. The two strategies constitute a challenge for dentistry that fulfills the successive stages of prevention.

2 Anatomopathology of the Carious Dentin: The Basis of ART Therapy

Carious tissue includes two layers. The first outer layer is named **infected dentin**. It contains denatured fragmented collagen fibers, numerous bacteria colonies, and food debris. The inner layer is called **affected dentin** and is located under the infected layer [3, 4]. Its consistency is harder than the soft demineralized layer. The collagen fibrils are not denatured. The objective of ART is to remove the infected dentin, and seal the cavity

with an adhesive material, promoting a favorable environment for the inner dentin which may heal. Adhesive properties of biomaterials play role in this process. After some time the mineral level return to a normal percentage in the deep layer, near the sound dentin composition. It is clear that the efficient treatment of the lesion implies the preservation of the sclerotic zone, allowing ions diffusion in the partially demineralized carious tissue, which keep the potential for remineralization.

In continuity with the enamel early lesion, shown to heal spontaneously, the early carious lesion includes microbial invasion (or necrotic zone), crossing the dentino-enamel junction (DEJ), spreading along the DEJ. The active decay erodes the mantle dentin and progress in the deeper dentin layers, and if there is no therapy, the lesion reaches the dental pulp.

The **superficial dentin** is deeply altered (soft carious dentin, or decalcified layer), and collagen fibers are partially destroyed by endogenous metalloproteinases and exogenous bacterial proteases. Enzymes cleave the collagen fibrils into 1/4 and 3/4 segments. Cathepsin K cut both tooth helical C-and N-terminals, and remove the telopeptides from the collagen fibers. Cysteine cathepsin degrade type I collagen, laminin, fibronectin, and proteoglycans (Fig. 1). MMPs, MMP inhibitors, and cysteine cathepsins are co-distributed in dentin. They are both active, synergically. Once the cavity is directly exposed to bacteria, tubular invasion occurs and the infected dentin becomes the zone of destruction.

Active lesions differ from **arrested** dentinal caries by its degree of pigmentation. Viable bacteria within the tubules, and lower calcium content accompany the decrease in hardness of active lesions. In arrested caries, the lumens of the **sclerotic** layer are filled by non-apatitic mineralizations characterized by their crystallographic properties such as weddellite, whewellite, calcite, brushite, whitlockite, and octocalcium phosphate. The lumens of sclerotic dentin are filled with a dense calcified material. The intertubular zone is well mineralized, in continuity with the peritubular dentin. Reactionary and reparative

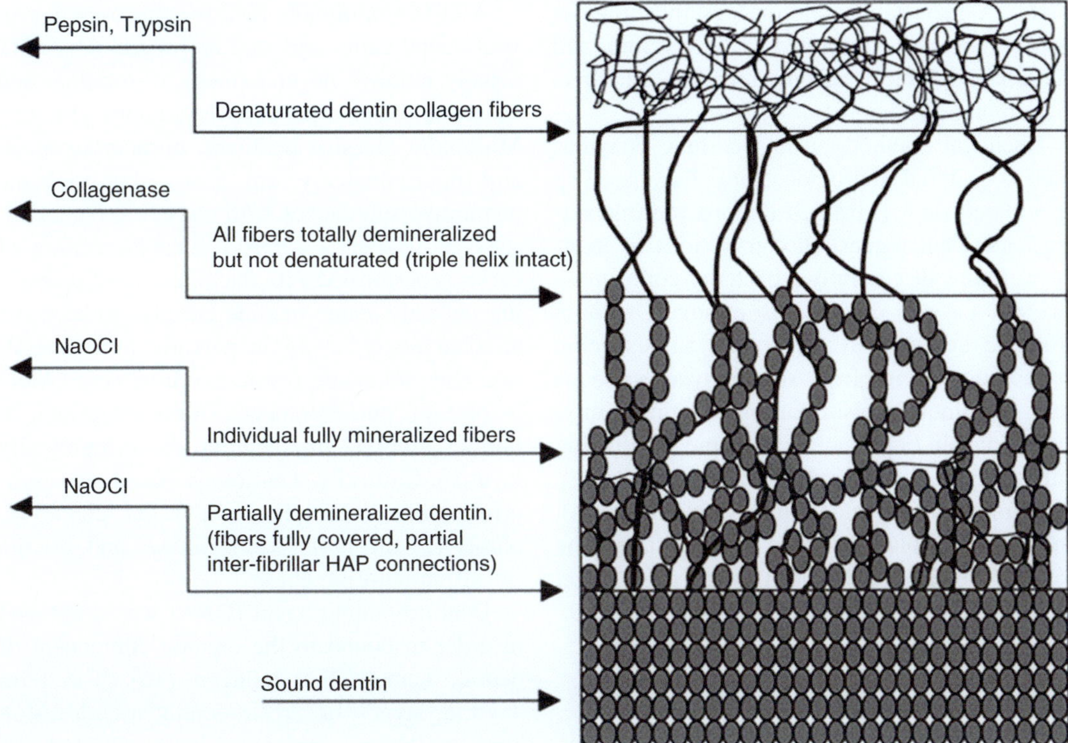

Fig. 1 Collagen degradation within the carious lesion [5, 6]

dentins are formed within the pulp, in front of the carious lesion.

With the occurrence of rapid lesion progression, the odontoblastic processes are destroyed without having contributed to tubular sclerosis. Dentin dead tracts are found. Some of these tubules are invaded by bacteria, and groups of tubules may coalesce to form liquefaction foci. Discoloration is one sign of carious lesions. Another sign is the softening of the tissues, including disintegration and eventually cavity formation. They are essential for differentiating active from arrested carious lesions, and moreover, the invaded layer from the affected layers [5].

In addition to mechanical removal of the soft carious dentin (using excavators, handpieces and—just to provide access—diamond-coated burs). Other methods include air-abrasion (bumbarding the tooth surface with aluminum oxide, or alumina particles, expecting to reduce the problems of heat and vibration). The methods so far used implicate also air-polishing ultrasonic instrumentation, and sono-abrasion.

Chemo-mechanical methods were more effective. The Caridex system (NMAB, GK-101E) was introduced and was further replaced by the Carisolv gel. Carisolv consists of two carboxymethylcellulose-based gels and a red gel containing erythrosine (added in order to make the gel visible during its use) and a second solution containing sodium hypochlorite (NaOCl— 0.5% w/v). The two are mixed in equal parts at room temperature before use and then applied, using hand instruments, onto the exposed dentine and left for 60 seconds prior to abrading away the softened dentine, leaving a hard, caries-free surface.

Current clinical techniques have been explored using lasers. They were successfully used in order to remove the carious dentine [7]. Casein phosphopeptide-amorphous calcium phosphate complexes (CCP-ACP) have the ability to stabilize high concentrations of calcium and phosphate in metastable solution, establishing an environment supersaturated with calcium and phosphate, inhibiting demineralization, and driving remineralization [6].

Chemical methods using certain enzymes such as bacterial Achromobacter collagenase [8], or stromelysin-1 (MMP-3) [9] provide interesting results but request shorter periods of treatment. Using successfully a bacterial collagenase the soft carious dentin was removed without affecting the sound layers. Pronase, a nonspecific proteolytic enzyme from streptomyces griseous helps to remove the soft carious dentin. A mixture of papain (a proteolytic enzyme eliminating only the partially degraded collagen molecule), chloramine (disinfectant inactivating bacteria), and toluidine blue provided good results. The name of the gel is Papacarie, a chemo-mechanical caries removal agent [10]

2.1 Minimal Intervention Dentistry (MID) and/or Atraumatic Restorative Treatment (ART)

The concept of minimal intervention dentistry (MID) is based on all the factors that affect the onset and progression of the disease. It integrates prevention and treatment. The field of minimal intervention dentistry is wide, including the detection of lesions as early as possible, the identification of risk factors (risk assessment), the implementation of preventive strategies, and health education for the patient [11]. Atraumatic Restorative Treatment (ART) concern mainly the minimum intervention dentistry (MID) [12, 13]. In practice, glass-ionomer cements (GIC) are the most used material, with the advantage that the GIC has a delayed setting reaction that allows handling the material before it is completely set.

The term "modified ART" refers to the fact that ART approach has been carried out in places where traditional dental equipment is not available. Therefore, "modification" is most often associated with the use of rotary equipment: to drill and open the tooth cavity, followed by the normal ART procedure.

ART is a minimally invasive approach to prevent dental caries and stop its progression. ART usually requires no unaesthetic restoration, and causes minimal discomfort to patients [14, 15]. Minimally invasive dentistry, ultraconservative, and micro-dentistry are terms that embrace restorative approaches with respect to dental tissues and patient's comfort. The excavation of caries is performed with the objective of preserving not only sound dentine but also to keep the affected dentin having the potential to remineralize. The atraumatic restorative treatment (ART) is part of our therapeutic armamentarium. It implies minimal intervention and is minimally invasive. Clinically, a cariology-based plan comprises three main phases: (1) the diagnostic phase, (2) the prophylactic phase, and (3) the (recall) monitoring phase.

Dentin bonding agent (DBA) was developed in order to bound to the organic component of dentin, namely the collagen [16]. The term "hybrid layer" or "resin-dentin interdiffusion zone" or "resin-impregnated layer" referred to a mechanism of bonding of resin-based DBAs via the formation of an hybrid layer [17].

The effectiveness of ART restorations is assessed by their survival. The most recent meta-analyses on the performance of ART restorations concluded that:

- ART using high-viscosity glass-ionomer can safely be used in single-surface cavities in both primary and permanent posterior tooth;
- ART using high-viscosity glass-ionomer cannot be routinely used in multiple-surface cavities in primary posterior tooth;
- Insufficient information is available for conclusions about ART restorations in multiple-surfaces in permanent posterior teeth, and in anterior teeth in both dentitions [18].

It was shown that bacteria remain present after complete hand excavation within the tubuli of affected dentin. The potential caries risk due to the remaining bacteria can be successfully controlled by reducing bacteria and through remineralization of the affected layer. Caries activity can be decreased through effective nutrient deprivation, and sealing the cavity using filling-materials that chemically bond to the cavity walls and which contribute to the remineralization of affected dentin, through longtime fluoride and other ions incorporation [15].

2.2 ART Failures

Clinical factors responsible for ART failures implicate the restorative biomaterial, the operator and technical factors. The prevention and management of ART failures includes first a correct clinical indication, and secondly, the repair of failed restorations.

The classification of sites follows the surface areas on which more frequently caries occurs.

- Site 1: pits and fissures (occlusal and other smooth tooth surfaces),
- Site 2: contact area between two adjacent teeth,
- Site 3: cervical area in contact with gingival tissues,

The main reason for clinical ART failures is related to operator skills and performance [19]. Failures results usually from restoration losses and fractures [20].

Minimal intervention dentistry is part of pediatric dentistry. General dental practice may adopt protocols that will promote early preventive visits and guidance rather than waiting for the need of restorative treatment [21].

2.3 Conclusions: What ART Provide to Vulnerable Patients?

It has been shown that the fluoridation of water reduced the prevalence of dentine lesions by approximately 50%. The main long-term action of fluoride is retarding the progression of carious lesions, rather than prevention of caries development. It can be concluded that only the "infected" ("outer carious") dentin layer needs to be removed, whereas the "affected" ("inner carious" and partially "demineralized") dentin should remain, even with bacteria within a small number of tubules. This demineralized dentin will remineralize under a well-sealed restoration. A new area for Atraumatic Restorative Treatment (ART) was instored some years ago and Black's cavities were relegated to the history of dental treatments. There are at least three aspects of caries therapies, including: (1) early caries detection and caries risk assessment; (2) remineralization of partially demineralized dentine and (3) optimal caries-preventive measures. ART involves tissue saving and cheap expenses. Economically ART favors weak the oral health in underdeveloped countries.

3 Etiopathology and Treatment of Gingival and Periodontal Tissues: From Gingivitis to Periodontitis

Free and attached gingiva constitute a "classical" division of clinically "normal" gingiva. Reference is usually given to the orange peel appearance due to numerous regularly distributed small depressions. Only the attached gingiva is stippled. This is due to the functional adaptation to mechanical impacts of collagen fibers of the lamina propria. The gingival grove underline the division between the free and attached gingiva. The free gingiva is that portion of the gingiva which surrounds the tooth and is separated from it by the gingival sulcus (Fig. 2). It may be subdivided into a region facing the tooth, another forming the crest of the gingiva and a domain facing the oral cavity. The attached gingiva is the region attached to the tooth. It includes the epithelium and its variations of component (stratum basale and suprabasale, stratum spinosum, stratum granulosum (dark membrane-coating granules). The superficial stratum corneum is composed either by ortho or parakeratinized layers and/or non-keratinized forms.

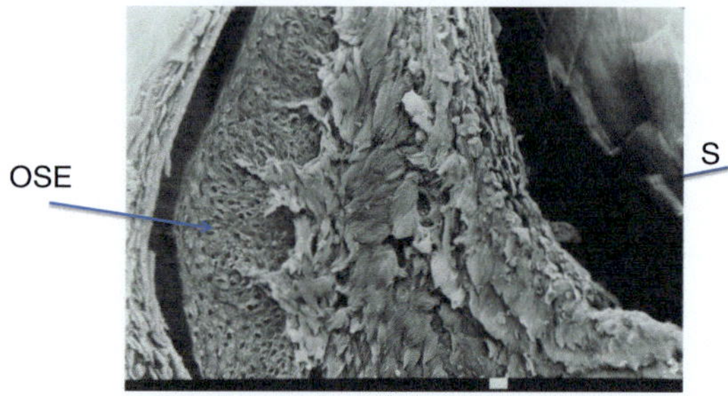

Fig. 2 Gingiva of rat's molar, *OSE* outer sulcular epithelium, S = sulcus (keratinized inner and outer sulcus)

3.1 Non-keratinocyte Cells Present in the Gingiva and in the Skin

Melanocytes and **Langerhans cells** are located between basal and spinous cells layers. Langerhans cells present antigen in the epidermis. In the connective tissue also called lamina propria, division is made between the papillary layer, and the reticular inner portion, attached to the alveolar bone. Between the inner sulcular epithelium and the teeth surface, a junctional epithelium is implicated in adhesion of keratinocytes to the cementum/dentin surface of the tooth [22].

Monocyte/macrophage system undergo significant changes in phenotype and functional properties (adherence, antigen presentation, and cytotoxicity) [23].

Mast cells are derived from hematopoietic precursors that arise in the bone marrow and circulate in the blood. In murine rodents, this process results in at least two distinct mast cell populations: the connective tissue-type mast cells (CTMC) and the mucosal mast cells (MMC) which occur in the mucosa of the gastro intestinal tract [24].

Cytoplasmic antigens of three different specificities are expressed in the epidermis. They differ by their location in distinct layers. One type is present in all epidermal cells, another in the superficial layers, and the third only in basal cells, suggesting involvement in differentiation and heterogeneity of the cells inside gingiva [25].

Periodontal diseases have been classified as follows (gingival and periodontitis):

- Gingivitis associated with dental plaque, with or without contributing factors,
- Gingival diseases modified by systemic factors, by medications, and malnutrition,
- Non-plaque induced gingival lesions,
- Chronic periodontitis,
- Aggressive periodontitis,
- Periodontitis as manifestation of systemic diseases,
- Necrotizing periodontal disease,
- Periodontal abscesses and development of acquired deformities.

3.2 Periodontal Diseases: Gingivitis and Periodontitis

Gingivitis, which affects the gums and coronal junctional epithelium, is characterized by loss of connective tissue attachment. Therefore, irreversible lesions are caused by a persistent inflammatory response promoted by alteration of the periodontal biofilm [26]. Gingivitis, the mildest form of periodontal disease, is a rapidly inducible and reversible inflammatory affection of the gingiva, mainly caused by accumulation of bacterial biofilm.

Attempts to identify periodontal diseases in relation to aetiology, pathogenesis and treatment were not totally successful. Gingivitis is caused by the bacterial biofilm (dental plaque) that accumulates on tooth adjacent to the gingiva. Gingivitis is reversible and prevention should eradicate the disease at this early stage. Periodontitis implies a loss of connecting tissue and bone support. The colonization of tooth surface is established in close contact with the gingival margin (gingival crevices), attachment loss, and subgingival pockets formation. In addition, genetic and environmental factors contribute to teeth loss.

Common forms of periodontal disease have been associated with adverse pregnancy outcomes, cardiovascular disease, stroke, pulmonary disease, and diabetes, but the causal relations have not been established. Prevention and treatment are aimed at controlling the bacterial biofilm and other risk factors, arresting progressive disease, and restoring lost tooth support [27].

These diseases may be of developmental, inflammatory, traumatic, neoplastic, genetic, or metabolic origin. Nutritional deficiency, osteoporosis, diabetes type 2 (patients at risk for periodontitis and in addition retinopathy, nephropathy, neuropathy, and macro- vascular diseases). They may also be implicated in the periodontal association with systemic diseases: preterm birth, cardiovascular disease, and stroke. Severe periodontitis was associated with an increased intima media thickening. The relation between periodontal health and diabetes has been described as bidirectional. Pulmonary disease may be associated with periodontal disease. Elimination of inflammation remains a critical objective of periodontal therapy.

Gingivitis is a risk factor in periodontal disease [28]. Various stages of gingivitis may be characterized prior to the progression toward periodontitis. Severe periodontitis affects over 11% of adults and has systemic inflammatory consequences.

Primary prevention of periodontitis is achieved by preventing gingivitis via four approaches.

Plaque control improve gingival inflammation and lower plaque scores. Toothbrushes, flossing, and interdental brushes used at interproximal area are necessary. Brushing should be used at least twice a day for 2 min with a fluoridated dentifrice. Local or systemic anti-inflammatory agents may also interfere in the etiopathogeny of the disease [29].

Calculus (tartar) may form from calcification of plaque above or below the gum line, and plaque exacerbates inflammatory processes. The inflammatory reaction is associated with the progressive loss of periodontal ligament and alveolar bone, and as a consequence, mobility and loss of teeth.

3.3　How to Prevent Periodontal Diseases for Vulnerable Patients?

In many developing countries, poor general health are associated with compromised host defenses, restricted access to dental care, and inadequate oral hygiene with high occurrence of gingivitis and periodontitis. In the high-risk areas, the population-based prevention programs aimed at self-care education and health promotion should be less cost effective. In this regard, WHO recently issued a policy framework for oral health promotion that addresses environmental, economical, social, and behavioral causes of periodontal disease.

Toothbrushing, the use of dental floss, and other devices to remove bacterial plaque from the teeth are the most common ways of disrupting or removing the biofilm from teeth. Although these methods are effective if used every day, they require motivation and dexterity. Mouthwashes and dentifrices containing antibacterial drugs have been used as adjuncts for controlling the biofilm. Treatment for gingivitis should re-establish periodontal health, arrest of the progression of disease, prevent the recurrence of disease, and preserve the dentition in a state of health, comfort, and function. This goal can be accomplished by various nonsurgical and surgical therapies, depending on the specific treatment objective [27].

3.4　Periodontal Therapies

Nonsurgical therapies include mechanical instrumentation, ultrasonic debridement, supragingival and/or subgingival irrigation, root planning, local drug delivery (topical antiseptics treatments with 10% povidone-iodine applied subgingivally and 0.1% sodium hypochlorite solution), 4% chlorhexidine mouth rinse, administration of systemic or local antibiotics (amoxicillin-metronidazole, ciprofloxacin-tetracyclines, doxycycline, penicillins, ofloxacin, clindamycin, minocycline). A commercially available bio-absorbable chip containing 2.5 mg of chlorhexidine in a cross linked hydrolyzed gelatin matrix (Perio Chip) was developed and shown to reduce the probing depths.

In addition, ozone therapy, hyaluronan, omega-3 fatty acids, lasers membrane, and grafting materials were used according to the type of periodontal defect treated (i.e., supra-alveolar defects, intrabony, furcation, and fenestration defects) [30]. The efficacity of bisphosphonate therapy as an adjunct to scaling and root planning (SRP) was confirmed. Research suggests that bisphosphonates not only inhibit osteoclast-mediated bone resorption, but also induce osteoblast cells to promote early bone formation.

Manual and ultrasonic debridement can be used to treat most patients with mild-to-moderate chronic periodontitis. An effective anti-carious fluoride treatment should constitute an integrated part of periodontal therapy [31, 32].

Scaling and root planning combined with gingival curettage was a common procedure for periodontal therapy. Gingival curettage, defined as the removal, by means of a curette, of the inner surface of the soft-tissue wall of the pocket, was performed in order to promote new attachment leading to pocket depth reduction.

The nonsurgical periodontal treatment remains the gold standard for managing the periodontal patients. Manual and ultrasonic débridement can be used to treat most patients with mild-to-moderate chronic periodontitis. Patients who do not practice optimal plaque control can enhance their personal hygiene procedures by using supragingival irrigation providing reduction of inflammation, pocket depth reduction, and clinical attachment gain [33].

Surgical Periodontal Therapy In situations where signs of inflammation persist, surgical therapy may be indicated. The predominant technique being excision of the diseased gingival tissue. Pocket elimination then became the main objective of periodontal therapy, and the gingivectomy or apically positioned flap procedures were commonly performed to eliminate the periodontal pocket and allow access to the root surface for scaling and oral hygiene procedures. Flap surgery is indicated with a probing depth of ‡ 5.4 mm, while between 2.9 mm and 5.4 mm nonsurgical therapy is preferred.

Local Drug Delivery Both scaling and root planning alone, and scaling and root planning combined with a flap procedure are effective methods for the treatment of chronic periodontitis, in terms of attachment gain and reduction in gingival inflammation The results of enamel matrix derivative (EMD) *therapy* have shown that EMD (EMDOGAIN) positively influences periodontal wound healing [34]. Mechanical therapy is effective for the majority of patients with mild-to-moderate chronic periodontitis. Ultrasonic débridement may result in less chair time and operator fatigue than does manual instrumentation. Studies have indicated that supragingival irrigation enhanced the effects of tooth brushing and reduced gingival inflammation in patients who did not perform good oral hygiene.

Other methods are more expensive. Antibiotics may be appropriate for certain medically compromised patients. A combination of drugs (amoxicillin with clavulanic acid, and ciprofloxacin) may be efficient. Collagenase inhibitor have also been used contributing to some positive results.

4   Conclusions

Most patients with mild-to-moderate chronic periodontitis respond to nonsurgical therapy, however, some patients require surgical therapy. Antibiotics should be reserved for patients who do not respond to conventional treatment [33]. For vulnerable patients, nonsurgical treatment limited to the treatment of gingivitis via scaling and root planning may pave the way of prevention measures, and upgrade preventive and public health dentistry.

References

1. Black GV. A work on operative dentistry; the technical procedures in filling teeth. Chicago: Medico-Dental Publishing Company; 1917.
2. Frencken JE, Leal SC, Navarro MF. Twenty-five-year atraumatic restorative treatment (ART) approach: a comprehensive overview. Clin Oral Invest. 2012;16:1337–46.
3. Fusayama T. New concepts in operative dentistry: differentiating two layers of carious dentin and using an adhesive resin. Chicago: Quintessence Publishing; 1980. p. 13–58.
4. Ogawa K, Yamashita Y, Ichijo T, Fusayama T. The ultrastructure and hardness of the transparent layer of human carious dentin. J Dent Res. 1983;62:7–10.
5. Goldberg M. Superficial and deep carious lesions. In: Goldberg M, editor. Understanding dental caries; 2016. p. 85–96.
6. Shen P, Cai F, Nowicki A, Vincent J, Reynolds EC. Remineralization of enamel subsurface lesions by sugar-free chewing gum containing casein phosphopeptide-amorphous calcium phosphate. J Dent Res. 2001;80(12):2066–70.
7. Banerjee A, Watson TF, Kidd EAM. Dentin caries excavation: a review of current clinical techniques. Br Dental J. 2000;188:476–82.
8. Goldberg M, Keil B. Action of a bacterial achromobacter collagenase on the soft carious dentine: an in vitro study with the scanning electron microscope. J Biol Buccale. 1989;17:269–74.
9. Boukpessi MS, Camoin L, TenCate JM, Goldberg M, Chaussain-Miller C. The effect of stromelysin-1(MMP-1) on non-collagenous extracellular matrix proteins of demineralized dentin and the adhesive properties of restorative resins. Biomaterials. 2008;29(33):4367–73.
10. Jain K, Bardia A, Geetha S, Goel A. Papacarie: a chemomechanical caries removal agent. IJSS Case Rep Rec. 2015;1(9):57–60.
11. Featherstone JDB, Doméjean S. Minimal intervention dentistry: part 1. From 'compulsive' restoration dentistry to rational therapeutic strategies. Br Dent J. 2012;213(9):441–5.
12. Frencken JE, van Amerongen WE. The atraumatic restorative treatment approach. In: Fejerskov O, Kidd E, Bente N, editors. Dental caries: the disease and its clinical management. 2nd ed. Oxford: Blackwell Munksgaard; 2008. p. 427–42.
13. Frencken Jo E, Leal SC. The correct use of the ART approach. J Appl Oral Sci. 2010;18(1):1–4.
14. Holmgren CJ, Roux D, Doméjean S. Minimal intervention dentistry: part 5. Atraumatic restorative treatment (ART)- a minimum intervention and minimally invasive approach for the management of dental caries. Br Dent J. 2013;214(1):11–8.
15. Frencken JE. The state-of-the-ART of ART restorations. Dent Update. 2014;41:218–24.
16. Nakabayashi N, Takarada K. Effect of HEMA on bonding to dentin. Dent Mater. 1992;8(2):125–30.
17. Tyas MJ, Burrow MF. Adhesive restorative materials: a review. Aust Dent J. 2004;49(3):112–21.
18. Francken JE, Holmgren CJ. Caries management through the Atraumatic Restorative Treatment (ART) approach and glass-ionomer update 2013. Braz Oral Res. 2014;28(1):1–4.
19. Mickenautsch S, Grossman E. Atraumatic Restorative Treatment (ART)- factors affecting success. J Appl Oral Sci. 2006;14:34–6.
20. Smales RJ, Yip H-K. The atraumatic restorative treatment (ART) approach for primary teeth: review of literature. Pediatr Dent. 2000;22:294–8.
21. Ramos-Gomez FJ, Crystal YO, Domejean S, Featherstone JDB. Minimal intervention dentistry: part 3. Paediatric dental care- prevention and management protocols using caries risk assessement for infants and young children. Br Dent J. 2012;213:501–8.
22. Bernimoulin J-P, Schroder HE. Quantitative electron microscopic analysis of the epithelium of normal human alveolar mucosa. Cell Tissue Res. 1977;180:383–401.
23. Weber-Matthiesen K, Sterry W. Organisation of the monocyte/macrophage system of normal human skin. J Invest Dermatol. 1990;95:83–9.
24. Tsai M, Shih L-S, Newlands GFJ, Takeishi T, Langley KE, Zsebo K, Miller HR, Geissier EN, Gali SJ. The rat c-kit ligand, stem cell factor, induces the development of connective tissue-type and mucosal mast cells in vivo. Analysis by anatomical distribution, histochemistry, and protease phenotype. J Experim Med. 1991;174(1):125–31.
25. Bystryn J-C, Nash M, Robins P. Epidermal cytoplasmic antigens: II. Concurrent presence of antigens of different specificities in normal human skin. J Invest Dermatol. 1978;71(2):110–3.
26. Scapoli L, Girardi A, Palmieri A, Martinelli M, Cura F, Lauritano D, Carinci F. Quantitative analysis of periodontal pathogens in periodontitis and gingivitis. J Biol Regulat Homeost Agents. 2015;29(3):101–10.
27. Pihlstrom BL, Michlowiicz BS, Johnson NW. Periodontal diseases. Lancet. 2005;366(Issue 9499):1809–20.
28. Lang NP, Schätzle MA, Löe H. Gingivitis as a risk factor in periodontal diseas. J Clin Periodontol. 2009;36(s10):3–9.
29. Chapple ILC, Van der Weijden F, Doerfer C, Herrera D, Shapira L, Polak D, et al. Primary prevention of periodontitis: managing gingivitis. J Clin Periodontol. 2015;42:S71–6.
30. Sculean A, Nikolidakis D, Schwarz F. Regeneration of periodontal tissue: combinations of barrier membranes and grafting materials- biological foundation and preclinical evidence: a systematic review. J Clin Periodontol. 2008;35(s8):106–16.
31. Slots J. Selection of antimicrobial agents in periodontal therapy. J Periodont Res. 2002;37:389–98.

32. Slots J. Low-cost periodontal therapy. Periodontol. 2012;60(1):110–37.
33. Greenstein G. Nonsurgical periodontal therapy in 2000: a literature review. JADA. 2000;131:1580–92.
34. Sculean A, Schwartz F, Becker J, Brecx M. The application of an enamel matrix protein derivative (Emdogain ®) in regenerative periodontal therapy: a review. Med Princ Pract. 2007;16:167–80.
35. Heitz-Mayfield LJA, Lang NP. Surgical and non-surgical periodontal therapy. Learned and unlearned concepts. Periodontology. 2000;2013(62):218–31.

Dental Neglect

Joseph Shapira

Young children are depend on their parents and caregivers to maintain their proper oral health. This includes managing of oral hygiene, healthy diet, and seeking for a treatment when needed. Untreated dental disease can have a significant adverse impact on the health, well-being, and quality of life of the child [1, 2].

The concept of Dental Neglect is generally defined as the inability to address basic oral health needs of children, "is willful failure of parent or guardian to seek and follow through with treatment necessary to ensure a level of oral health essential for adequate function and freedom from pain and infection" [3]. The Royal College of Paediatrics and Child Health [4], add and emphasize "the persistent failure to meet a child's basic oral health needs, which is likely to result in the serious impairment of the child's oral and general health and growth & development" which are significantly impaired.

Dental neglect can cause infections and swelling in the mouth, and nearby areas, to the risk of life, especially in very young children who require general anesthesia for the removal of infected carious teeth, this is a procedure that is never without risk [5].

Untreated dental caries can cause pain in the mouth area that will cause eating disorders and improper nutrition [6], because the child swallows food instead of chewing it, weight loss [2] and improper physical development, sleep disturbances, and interference with performance at school [7]. In addition, extensive destruction of the child's teeth can cause damage to the child's speech and pronunciation of the words and impair the aesthetics of the child's mouth and face [8]. Interruptions such as these can damage the child's communication with the world of children and adults around him and, no less, his self-image. In addition to this, when this condition of neglect persists for a long time, there may be disturbances in learning, inability to concentrate, and a general decline in the quality of his life [9].

From a purely dental viewpoint, untreated caries in the primary teeth had been 2.2 times more likely to have a enamel defect in their succeeding permanent teeth and where the primary tooth had been lost for a reason such as extraction due to caries/abscess, the permanent tooth was associated with a 5.0 times increased odds of having a enamel opacity [10]. In addition, infections caused by lack of treatment of the primary teeth can lead to abscess around and between their roots and consequently developmental damage in the permanent teeth that follow them [3, 8, 11].

J. Shapira (✉)
Department of Pediatric Dentistry, The Hebrew University-Hadassah School of Dental Medicine, Jerusalem, Israel

The Hebrew University-Hadassah School of Dental Medicine, Department of Pediatric Dentistry, Hadassah Medical Center, Jerusalem, Israel
e-mail: shapiraj@cc.huji.ac.il
JosephSha@ekmd.huji.ac.il

The oral characteristics of dental neglect include widespread caries in a large number of teeth, dental pain and, of course, the risk of regional oral infection due to non-treatment. Studies and surveys showed that children who were abused also had tooth decay at a higher rate than in other healthy children with the same age [12].

It is often difficult to distinguish between extensive cavities in children's teeth and what is called extensive caries due to dental neglect. There is no doubt that the definition of neglect can only be read **if the parent or guardian of the child is not working to allow the child to receive dental treatment or has stopped treatment for any reason** [11].

The "dental neglect" will then be considered as "child abuse" if the parent of a child is warned by a medical professional about the significance and severity of the child's dental condition and what should be done about it, and yet he is not working to change the situation [3, 8, 11]. The clinician should also determine whether dental services are readily available and accessible to the child when considering whether negligence has occurred [3].

For the possible reasons that may "justify" "dental neglect," one must consider the indifference of parents in a family with many children, low socioeconomic status, social isolation, and lack of appreciation for the importance of oral health in children and especially the possible idea that in any case, these "milk teeth" are soon shed [13]. The World Health Organization has stated that neglect has to be distinguished from circumstances of poverty, implying that neglect can only occur in cases where reasonable resources are available to the family or caregiver [14]. In countries, where the National Health Insurance Law provides eligibility for state-funded dental treatments, the economic factor is not a barrier or excuse for not bringing children to care for their teeth.

In Israel, for example, according to the National Health Insurance Law of 2010 [15] children up to the age of 18 are entitled to receive dental treatments as part of the health basket and with state funding. Therefore, the economic factor is not a barrier to the failure of children to take care of their teeth.

Dentists are strongly encouraged to collaborate with their local safeguarding/child protection team in order to ensure that prompt and appropriate referrals are made when concerns regarding dental neglect arise [8].

What are the characteristics of parents of children suffering from dental neglect [8, 11]:

1. Lack of basic oral health services such as brushing teeth on the one hand and encouraging nutrition that can cause tooth decay such as sweets, snacks, and sweetened beverages on the other hand.
2. Lack of cooperation with the dental guidelines and recommendations for the child's care. Because of fear of the dental environment as perceived either by the child or by the parent.
3. Inconsistent or logical explanations of the parent's questioning of the child situation and lack of perception of a need for dental care.
4. Hard parenting and over-control.
5. Suspicion of dental neglect bordering on abuse should be suspected when, in the parents' questioning, there is a dominant parent who does not allow the investigation of each parent separately.

1 Concluding Remarks

The difficult determination when does the present of dental disease equal parental/caregiver neglect is a sensitive one since the pediatric dentist' interest is the child health.

The point at which to consider a parent negligent and to begin intervention occurs only after the parent has been properly alerted by a health care professional about the nature and extent of the child's condition, the specific treatment needed, and the mechanism of accessing that treatment [16].

The dentist should be certain that the parents/caregivers understand the explanation of the disease and its implications and, when barriers to the needed care exist, attempt to assist the families in finding financial aid, transportation, or public facilities for needed services. If, despite these efforts the parents fail to obtain therapy, the case should be reported to appropriate child protective services [3, 17].

2 The Main Problems Concerning Dental Neglect and How to Resolve Them

The main problems in handling suspicion on dental neglect in the dental practice are the **identification** and the **establishing** of an adequate team collaboration between the practicing dentist and the local child protection of the welfare system.

Imagine that during the routine examination of the kindergartens, the examiners diagnosed the two cases before us:

2.1 Case 1

In this case (Fig. 1), the child was diagnosed as a "bottle syndrome baby" = ECC. In a routine check-up, the parent were asked to stop the habit and receive urgent treatment for the affected injured teeth, the parents obeyed and the child was treated to the satisfaction of everyone with no recurrence of tooth decay in the other teeth in a monitored follow-up check-up.

2.2 Case 2

Although the child was examined in the past, and the parents were then asked to take him to get care with only the upper incisors and the first molars having tooth decay (Fig. 2), they did stop the habit—of drinking sweet from a bottle at night while sleeping—but did not take the child for treatment due to their fear of general anesthesia at this young age.

Few months later, dental examination revealed (Fig. 3) that more teeth are involved with large caries lesions and the need for urgent care were explained to parents again. Considering the large amount of work needed and the difficult behavior problems of the child, the parents with the interventional aid of the teacher and kindergarten nurse, convinced at last the implementation of a comprehensive dental treatment under general anesthesia.

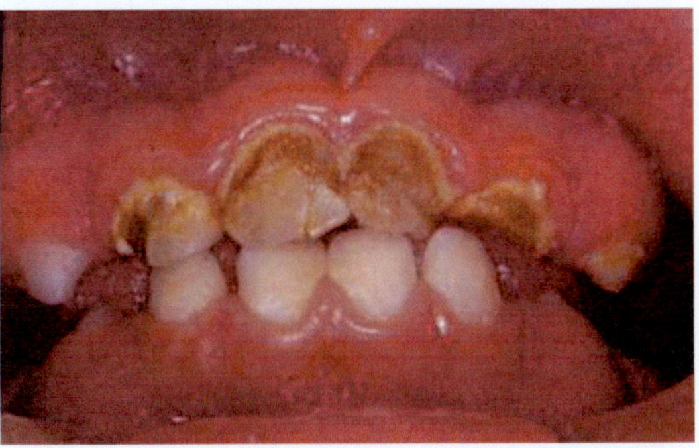

Fig. 1 "Baby bottle syndrome" = ECC. (This picture is the property of the Department of Pediatric Dentistry, Hebrew University—Hadassah School of dental Medicine, Jerusalem, Israel)

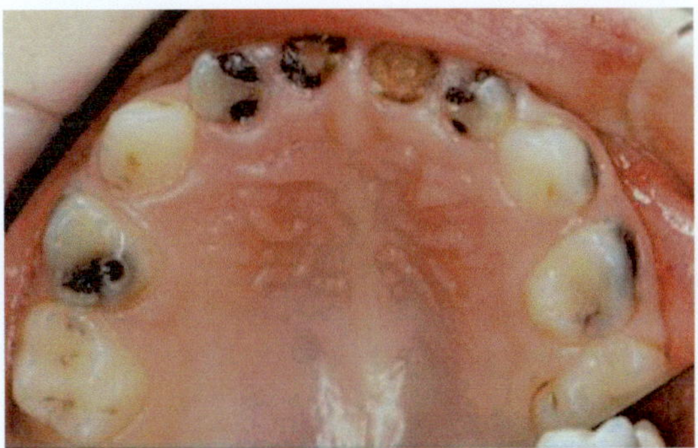

Fig. 2 Upper incisors and first molars with tooth decay after "baby bottle syndrome" = ECC. (This picture is the property of the Department of Pediatric Dentistry, Hebrew University—Hadassah School of dental Medicine, Jerusalem, Israel)

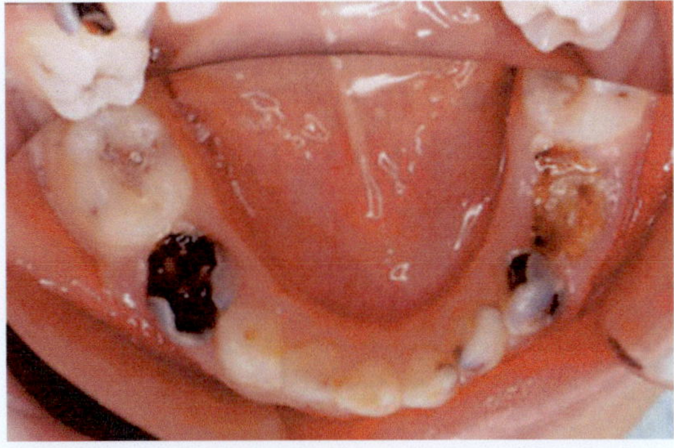

Fig. 3 Dental examination reveals large caries lesions in several teeth "baby bottle syndrome" = ECC. (This picture is the property of the Department of Pediatric Dentistry, Hebrew University—Hadassah School of dental Medicine, Jerusalem, Israel)

3 Conclusion

It is our responsibility to provide the family with appropriate friendly dental services, concerning many variables like age, behavior, risk that are convenient and meet the needs of children and families.

For this purpose, we need to be able to get advice about individual cases, by working closely together: dentist, teacher, and dental nurse in order to make decisions. This team should determine whether dental services are readily available and accessible to the child when considering whether negligence has occurred.

The children who are being neglected don't know that. It is therefore **our** responsibility to be alert. Intervention is not only the responsibility of a particular dentist, but rather is a shared public challenge.

References

1. Low W, Tan S, Schwartz S. The effect of severe caries on the quality of life in young children. Pediatr Dent. 1999;21:325–6.
2. Sheiham A. Dental caries affects body weight, growth and quality of life in preschool children. Br Dent J. 2006;201:625–6.
3. American Academy of Pediatric Dentistry: policies and guidelines. 2017. p. 177–9.
4. The Royal College of Paediatrics and Child Health (RCPCH). Child protection evidence – systematic review on dental neglect. 2017.
5. Kakounaki E, Tahmassebi JF, Fayle SA. Repeat general anaesthesia, a 6-year follow up. Int J Paediatr Dent. 2011;21:126–31.
6. Clark M, Locker D, Berall G, Pencharz P, Kenny DJ, Judd P. Malnourishment in a population of young children with severe early childhood caries. Pediatr Dent. 2006;28:254–9.
7. Blumenshine SL, Vann WFJ, Gizlice Z, Lee JY. Children's school performance: impact of general and oral health. J Public Health Dent. 2008;68:82–7.
8. The Royal College of Pediatrics and Child Health RCPCH. Child protection evidence-systemic review on dental neglect. 2017.
9. Arrow P. Child oral health-related quality of life (COHQoL), enamel defects of the first permanent molars and caries experience among children in Western Australia. Community Dent Health. 2013;30(3):183–8.
10. Broadbent JM, Thompson WM, William SM. Does caries in primary teeth predict enamel defects in permanent teeth? A longitudinal study. J Dent Res. 2005;84:260–4.
11. Bhatia S, et al. Characteristics of child dental neglect: a systematic review. J Dent. 2014;42:229–39.
12. Sillevis SH, de Leeuw J, de Vries T. Association between severe dental caries and child abuse and neglect. J Oral Maxillofac Surg. 2017;75:2304–6.
13. Campus G, Lumbau A, Sanna AM, et al. Oral health condition in an Italian preschool population. Eur J Paediatr Dent. 2004;5:86–91.
14. Krug EG, Dahlberg LL, Mercy JA, Zwi AB, Lozano R. World report on violence and health. Geneva: World Health Organization; 2002.
15. www.health.gov.il/Subjects/Dental_health/ChildrenDentalTreatmentsReform
16. California Society of Pediatric Dentists. Dental neglect: when to report. Calif Pediatric. 1989;1(Fall):31–2.
17. American Academy of Pediatrics. Oral and dental aspects of child abuse and neglect. Pediatrics. 1999;104:348–50.

The Vulnerable Patients Group: The Global Oral Health Concept

Akinboboye Bolanle Oyeyemi

1 Introduction

In November 2000 the FDI-World Dental Organization celebrated the 100th Anniversary. One century of an amazing development of the Dental discipline. At this opportunity the leaders begin to look of a new definition of the futures aims, and the strategies. In 2012 as result of the FDI resolution published an article entitled: FDI Vision 2020: shaping the future of Oral Health [1]. Recently in 2020 appear a new Journal: Journal of **Global** Oral Health a publication of the Academy of Dentistry International in conjunction with the NCD of the WHO [2].

There is no doubt that important steps are achieved, but the problem is if these information have reached the simple General Practitioners GP and What is he's profit for an improvement of the daily clinical work.

With the apparition of the pandemic COVID-19 the situation is going worst despite all the efforts of the legal authorities.

In fact the global aim imperatively concerns an adapted anamnesis and a selected treatment plane; for example there is a large consensus that neglected Periodontics problems are the reason of the loos of the majority of the teeth [3].

Finally, looking on number of articles there are no evaluation data on the efficiency of the presentation and the advises.

Therefore it seems necessary starting a follow-up in a number of different countries; Nigeria, Georgia, USA, Canada, Australia, Norway, and Sweden.

Many articles were published the last decade, from the FDI or from the ECG (European College of Gerontology); mainly dealing with Elderly. In the surveys the loss of teeth and the edentulous patients seem to be the focus of the research [4–6].

A side this very few is mentioned about the huge majority of vulnerable patients.

Therefore in this chapter we are trying to investigate the reasons for the barriers against a Global Oral Health Program. Were examined Articles concerning several of these countries [7].

A. B. Oyeyemi (✉)
Department of Restorative Dentistry, Faculty of
Dental Sciences, College of Medicine, University of
Lagos, Lagos, Nigeria

Different points were relevant such as:

- The Lack of an Oral health policy, about the participation in the burden of National or private insurances.
- Difficult access for education, and the Health facilities.
- Small possibilities to adapt the new technologies.

- Ignorance from a great part of the population about a basic preventive behavior.
- The incidence of the poverty factor in the creation of a neglected population [8].
- Lack of coordination between the Professional organization and the legal authorities [9].
- The outstanding help from the voluntary NGO [10] (Figs. 1 and 2).

	Germany	United Kingdom	Sweden	Switzerland	Finland	Israel	Georgia	USA	Australia
Edentulism	40.2%	57%	23%	26.8%	11%	61%	73.8%	50%	35%
Remaining teeth	20 29%	13	24.5	12	89% 1–32	35%	26–2%. 0–20	18–20	22
Partial restorations	Yes	Yes	Yes	Yes	Yes	Yes	Yes	38%	Yes
Caries	22%	23%	21%	29.3%	37.1%	27.2%	25.7%	6.3	36%
Periodontal	87%	60%	30%	45.1%	21.3%.%	67.4%	50%	20.7%	56%

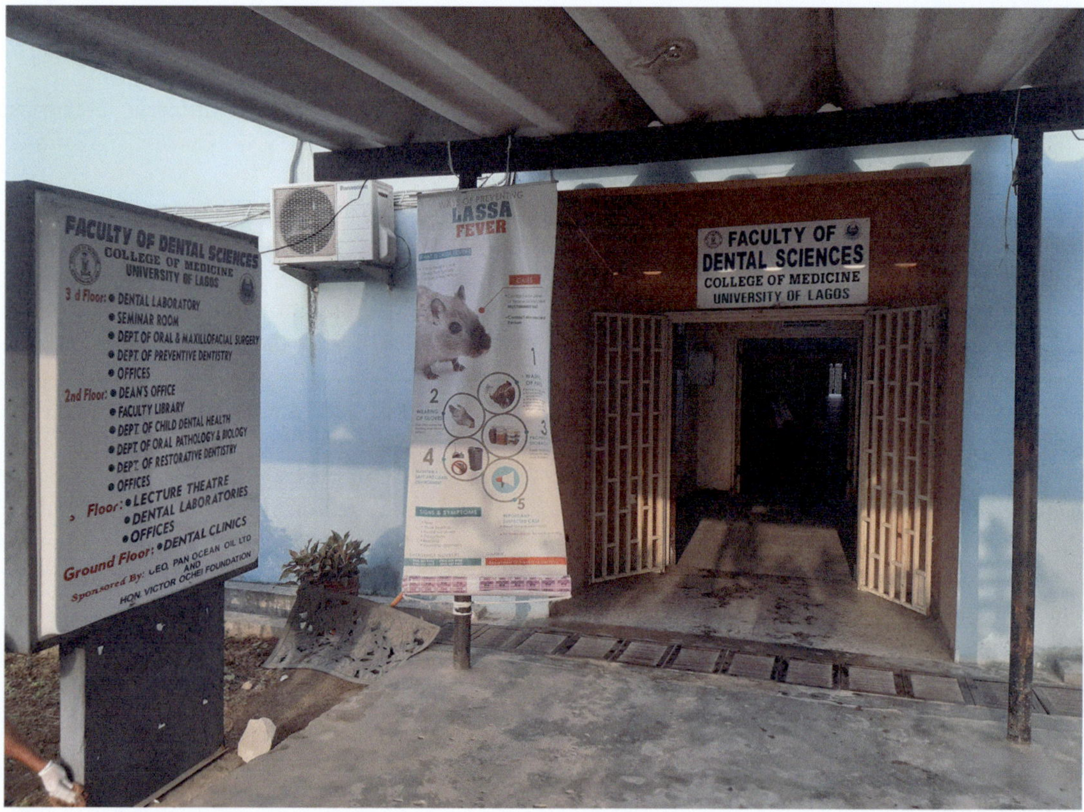

Fig. 1 The Dental Faculty in Lagos Nigeria

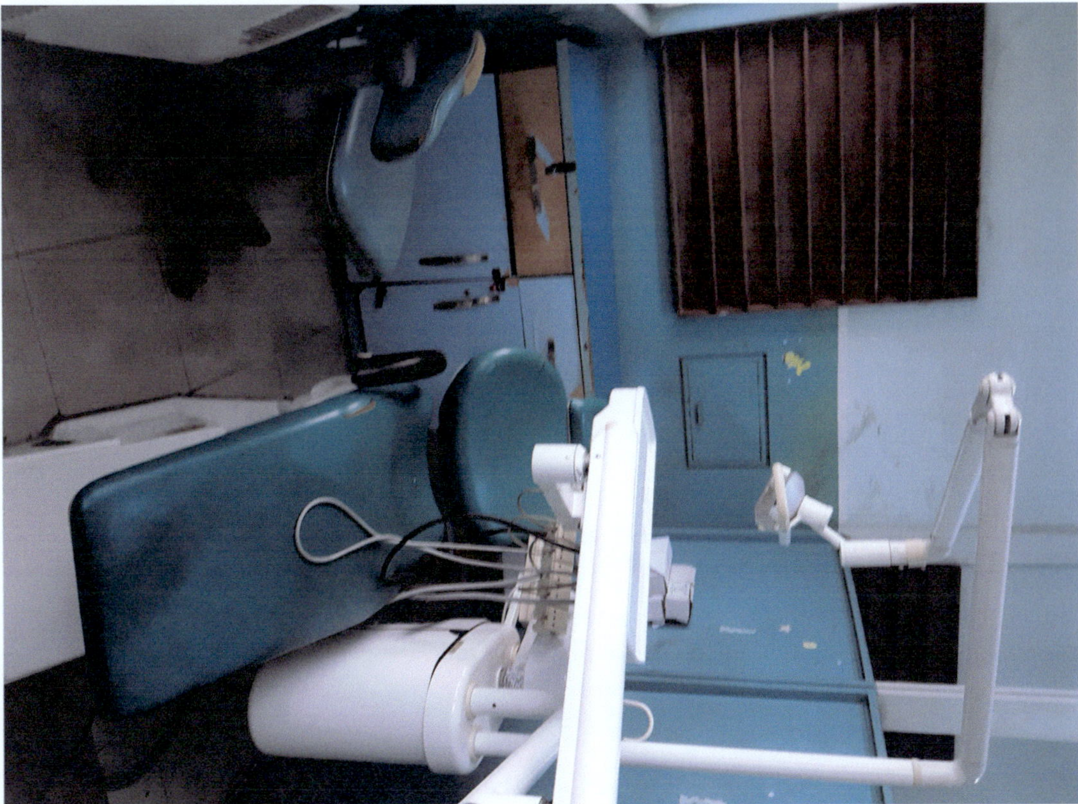

Fig. 2 The Dental clinic in Lagos Nigeria

1.1 Conclusion

This review underlined numerous facts.

1. There are serious differences between the countries.
2. The gap is independent from the number of the population, the superficies of the countries, the economic and social level, and the degree of poverty, the religion, and the climate. Anyway fees are an important barrier for dental treatments. Different systems of insurance; National or Private is a key issue.
3. There is an identity between countries which adapted a specific strategy. In fact launching a new terminology: Global Health is an official and necessary starting point. But since 2011, we are waiting for a practical education program. The General Practitioners are looking for an adapted strategy. Since the COVID-19 is introducing new complication, new issues will increase the number of vulnerable patients. Of course epidemiology and the traditional approach are essential, but do not offer solutions for the daily clinical issues. The philosophy of epidemiology is leading the Profession to ethical obligations [11].
4. In countries as Sweden and Finland a national consensus was leading on a Preventive track avoiding as result.

    The dramatic loss of teeth, and consequently important expenses for restorations and prosthetic devices.
5. In the European Union a great effort is done to introduce Oral Health for Elders and vulnerable people in the national challenges. (EPHA).
6. Nevertheless; few countries recently adapted a realistic policy. An FDI-ERO survey concerning 27 Countries pointed out. In 52%

there is a political/administrative agenda, but in 45% there are no initiatives.

For exception, Germany with the Collective group for Prevention, and in Slovenia with the Special skilled Teams.

During the last decades we are witness of an outstanding development of the African Countries.

Therefore, it will be instructive to learn about the conditions and The achievements in a country as Nigeria.

2 Overview of Dentistry in an African Country: Nigeria

The WHO estimated the population of elderly at 43 million in 2010, projected the population of elderly people in sub-Saharan Africa to reach 67 million by 2025 and 163 million by 2050. The population of those aged 65 years and above in Nigeria (which is one of the populous countries in sub Saharan Africa is 3.1% or 5.9 million of the total population of 191 million). This represents an increase of 600,000 during the 5-year period 2012–2017 (Population Reference Bureau 2012; National Council on Ageing, 2016). It is reported to be culturally and environmentally diverse (Population Reference Bureau 2012) with the fastest population growth, projected to become the third largest country in the world (National Council on Ageing 2016).

Aging is occurring despite contextual socio-economic hardship, general poverty, HIV/AIDS epidemic, and the rapid transformation of the traditional extended family structure [12]. The increase in older population has also attributed to the decline in fertility with a steady decrease from 1980 [13]. In 1980 the total registered fertility rate was 6.8 but in 2017 the total registered fertility rate was 5.5 [14–16]. Improved health and sanitary conditions have also been documented as one of the factors contributing to the rise of life expectancy.

There is a fast increase in the age group of 85 years and above (the old–old), the implication

is that there will be a challenge to meet the health, psychological, economic, and social well-being needs of the aging population especially with the breakdown of the traditionally extended family support [17]. Aging results in reduction in agility, frailty, increase risk of being disease prone and the outcome is discrimination, social isolation, dejection, and depression. There is oral health disparities and social inequality among the older age group and this is determined by various factors such as the location of the elderly whether urban or rural [18]. Other factors are the distribution of oral health services, accessibility, and utilization. The aging population are faced with changes in family dynamics, increased demand for healthcare services, increased economic burden, and increased functional dependence. All these factors pose challenges to effective delivery of health to the aging population.

2.1 Retirement

The statutory retirement age is 60, 70 years or 35 years of service (dependent on place of work) [19]. After retirement there is no regular income, as some have to rely on their pension or family members. There is an existing pension regulation scheme for the retired people but the implementation has not been a successful story. This is due to the fact that most of these population do not have sustainable standard of living in retirement and their benefits are not paid as at when due. There is also the problem of delayed or non-payment of pension entitlement, low standard of living as a result of disparity between pension and present rate of inflation. There is also migration from the urban to the rural part of the country as a result of difficulty in maintaining the standard of living [20]. These elderlies are vulnerable to economic hardship. These population continue to engage in menial jobs, manual works on farm resulting in health disorders, and physical exhaustion.

There is a connection between socioeconomic status and health outcomes. It is a belief that people with higher income and higher education take better advantage of health care services than those with lower income and lacking formal education; they are at a disadvantage in utilizing health care system [21].

2.2 Social Isolation

Another challenge faced with aging is social isolation, resulting in disconnection from family, friends, and community. Many of the community settings are not aging-friendly. A setting that is not designed for walk, or where there is poor transportation system (difficulty in driving and using public transportation) can contribute to lack of mobility for older adult and isolation. Older adults with disabilities such as physical disabilities may find it difficult walking to the nearest bus stop to get transportation. In this environment the public transport is mainly the buses, motorcycle, tricycle, and the least common is the train. These has negative impact on access to health care and quality of life [22]. Rural areas have higher incidence of poverty and less access to various community amenities [23, 24]. Isolation can also be chosen by an individual and some of them go into depression and the effect of isolation require attention, the policy makers can help in making policies that will help make community aging-friendly and reduce isolation in the elderly.

2.3 Policy for Older Adult

There is no proper policy for the elderly in our community. Many depend solely on the pension which in most cases does not come regularly. The retirement entitlement might be delayed for years. Those who do not work for government organization, work beyond the age of 60 years doing menial jobs and petty trading to get income to survive. Some become dependent on family and loved ones, with the increase risk of systemic diseases with aging, many are not able to afford health services because most of payment for health are done out of pocket. There is no proper insurance scheme for the older population and because of this many of the older population have their health failing both oral and general health. The shift in income from when in service and after retirement when there is no constant or regular income also have negative impact on the well-being of the older population. This also affect their social roles [25] and in some cases it symbolize the beginning of the end for the individual. The provision of social services such as income, security, healthcare, housing, and legal assistance can positively influence the well-being and health of the elderly [19]. There is lack of this social security in the nation for the older population. A policy was made in 1989 to provide a framework for protecting elderly persons from moral and material neglect and provide public assistance when necessary but there has been no effective implementation of such policy [19, 26]. In addition, there are also no policy changes in Nigeria [27] and the failure to regularly pay pension funds to retiree poses a critical threat to food, social, and national security [28]. Culturally, the elderly is respected in our communities. This should be inculcated by the government and the older population should be made priority in making any policy.

There are few geriatric departments in our teaching hospital and few specialists in the care of the elderly. Most of the elderly cannot afford the specialist so they visit the general practitioners in government hospitals. There is also the issue of lack of equipment and medical personnel with the advent of brain drain (doctors leaving the country in search of greener pastures). The geriatric homes are not so popular in this environment because of the cultural belief. However, there are few old people homes that cater for the elderly. There is the concern of the collapse of our cultural family structure that the elderly is cared for by their family [29]. The economic situation has also contributed to the lack of free medical treatment for the older population.

2.4 Policy Making and Implementation for Older Population

In terms of policy for the elderly the three arms of government should take care of the elderly: local, state, and federal level of government. Data base of the elderly in all community should be kept and a program should be initiated by government in which this database will serve as guide. More old people homes should also be established and private establishment and individuals should also buy into this program. Policy on regular payment of pension should be ensured, more specialist should be trained, geriatric courses should be incorporated into the medical and dental curriculum in our schools. Provision of social workers, easy transportation for older population and making the community aging friendly are some of the things that should be done to improve conditions of the elderly and ensure their well-being.

2.5 Conclusion

The major challenge with the face of rapid demographic change in Nigeria is poor policy implementation, lack of personnel to respond promptly to the needs of the aging population. The unsustainable economic growth is not also having positive impact on care of the elderly in addition to the collapse of the family structure and traditional care of the elderly. It is therefore necessary that policies be implemented that will focus on the issues facing the older population to improve their well-being and the quality of life.

References

1. FDI world Dental Federation. Leading the world to optimal oral health. Annual Report. 2019.
2. Herbst FA. Reflections on the social responsibility of the oral health profession particularly the Academy of Dentistry International. J Global Oral Health. 2019;2(2):07–12.
3. Ramsay SE, et al. Influence of poor oral heath on physical frailty: a population based cohort study of older British men. J Am Geriatr Soc. 2017;66(3):473–9. https://doi.org/10.1111/jgs.15175.1-18.
4. Stabholz A, et al. The reasons of tooth loss in geriatric patients attending two surgical clinics in Jerusalem. Gerodontology. 2008;14(2):83–8.
5. Baumgartner W, et al. Oral health and dental care of elderly adults dependent on care. Swiss Dent J. 2015;125(4):417–24.
6. Liu Y, et al. Social disparities in dentition status among American adults. Int Dent J. 2014;64(1):52–576.
7. Muller F, et al. What are the prevalence and incidence of tooth loss in the adult and elderly population in Europe ? Clin Oral Implants Res. 2007;18(3): 2–14.
8. A well established socio-economic gradient of Health. Correlation between poverty, social exclusion, and health inequalities between groups and countries. 2017. http://www.ocd.org/els/cope-divbide–europe-2017-background-report.pdf.
9. FDI-ERO WG Aging. A survey of 27 ERO member countries. Rusca: Ph. Swiss Dental Association; 2018.
10. Mersel A, et al. Oral rehabilitation for a geriatric population: a voluntary experience. Open J Stomatol. 2012;6-2:1–3.
11. Kaplan JM, Valles SA. Synthese. Springer; 2019. p. 1–10.
12. Adebanjoko A, Ugwuoke OW. Poverty and the challenges of insecurity to development. Eur Sci J. 2014;10(14):361–72.
13. Lee R, Mason A. Is low fertility really a problem? Population aging, dependency, and consumption. Science. 2014;10:229–34.
14. United Nations, Department of Economic and Social Affairs, Population Division. World population prospects: the 2015 revision. Key findings and advance tables (internet). New York: United Nations; 2015 (cited 2016 Aug 31). Report No.: ESA/P/WP.241. Available from: http://esa.un.org/unpd/wpp/publications/files/key_findings_wpp2015.pdf.
15. Population Reference Bureau. World population data sheet (2012). Washington, DC: Author; 2017.
16. United Nations Department of Economic and Social Affairs: Population Division. World population prospects: the 2015 revision. 2015. Retrieved from http://www.un.org/en/development/desa/publications/world-population-prospects-2015-revision.html.
17. Okoye UO. Family care-giving for ageing parents in Nigeria: gender differences, cultural imperatives and the role of education. Int J Educ Age. 2012;2(2):139–54.
18. Akinboboye BO, Ogunyemi AO, Ladi-Akinyemi TW. Orl health status and service utilization among a group of rural older Nigerians. African Journal Of Oral Health. 2018;8:24–31.
19. Oladeji D. Family care, social services, and living arrangements factors influencing psychosocial well-being of elderly from selected households in Ibadan, Nigeria. Educat Res Int. 2011;2011:1–6.
20. Akinboboye BO, Ogunyemi A. Treatment needs, demand, association of missing and replaced tooth

among older population in a rural setting. Nig J Dent Res. 2019;4:88–96.

21. Tanyi PL, Andre P, Mbah P, Tong K. Care of the elderly in Nigeria: implications for policy. Congent Soc Sci J. 2018;4(1):1.

22. Partners for Livable Communities, The National Association of Area Agencies on Ageing. A blueprint for action: developing a livable community for all ages. 2007. Retrieved from http://livable.org/storage/documents/reports/AIP/blueprint4actionsinglepages.pdf.

23. Fonchingong CC. Firming up institutional policy for deprived elderly in Cameroon: policy for deprived elderly in Cameroon. Polit Policy. 2014;42(6):948–80. https://doi.org/10.1111/polp.12101.

24. Snedeker L. Ageing and isolation – causes and impacts. Soc Work Today. 2017;17(1):24.

25. Kaplan DB, Berkman BJ. Effects of life transitions on the elderly. 2016. Retrieved from https://www.merckmanuals.com/professional/geriatrics/social-issues-in-the-elderly/effects-of-life-transitions-on-the-elderly.

26. Abdulkadir RI, Abdullah NA, Wong W. Dividend payment behaviour and its determinants: the Nigerian evidence. Afr Dev Rev. 2016;28:55–63.

27. Mudiare PE. Abuse of the aged in Nigeria: elders also cry. Am Int J Contemp Res. 2013;3(9):79–87.

28. Ajomale O. Country report: ageing in Nigeria—current state, social and economic implications. Summer newsletter of the research committee (RC11) of the sociology of aging of the International Sociological Association (ISA). 2007. p. 15–20.

29. Okoye UO, Asa SS. Caregiving and stress: experience of people taking care of elderly relations in South-Eastern Nigeria. Arts Soc Sci J. 2011;29:1–9.

30. The World Bank. Nigeria (Internet). Washington DC: The World Bank; 2015. http://data.worldbank.org/country/nigeria.

The TMJ Troubles and Their Nutritional Consequences

Marzia Segù

Let food be thy medicine

– attributed to Hippocrates

1 Impact of Painful TMD on Eating and Nutritional Status

TMDs are considered the most common cause of orofacial pain of nondental origin and are currently included within the musculoskeletal disorders.

TMD patients experienced impaired food intake ability [1] and discomfort when eating [2].

The symptoms are varied but are likely to affect the choice, intake, and enjoyment of food.

Pain is most frequently reported in the TMJ and is often linked to chewing actions, thus causing patients to experience **difficulty chewing some foods** and to **take longer to finish meals. This situation is also deteriorating the neglected people's nutrition.**

All conditions involving orofacial pain can (like any systemic condition, chronic or otherwise) have some impact on quality of life (QoL), where QoL is understood as an individual's degree of well-being linked both to subjective (personality traits) and objective factors (socioeconomic conditions, social relations, health, and working environment), and that it may even do so to an extent that results in various forms of social and psychological deprivation.

Quality of life assessment is one of the areas identified by the WHO as crucial for achieving "health for all," and in this context, surveys and questionnaires are a fundamental means of collecting data.

The Oral Health Impact Profile questionnaire (OHIP) is currently the instrument able to give us the most complete picture of the consequences of oral disorders and conditions [3].

It was formulated using methods similar to those used in the construction of the sickness impact profile (SIP), which was designed for the study of chronic disorders. The most important phase was the planning of a series of interviews and their subsequent administration to a heterogeneous sample of dental patients in order to gather information on the fundamental characteristics of oral disorders and their ability to reduce a patient's functional capacity. Since these interviews yielded at least as many as 535 important statements describing the influence of oral conditions on daily life, the material was reprocessed. This step resulted in the definitive formulation of 49 questions, divided, by content, into seven separate sections: functional limitation, physical pain, psychological discomfort, physical disabil-

M. Segù (✉)
University of Parma, Department of Medicine and Surgery, Parma, Italy
e-mail: marzia.segu@unipr.it

© The Author(s), under exclusive license to Springer Nature Switzerland AG 2022
A. Mersel (ed.), *Treatment Dilemmas for Vulnerable Patients in Oral Health*,
https://doi.org/10.1007/978-3-031-08435-5_5

ity, psychological disability, social disability, and handicap. The battery of 49 questions can be administered by interviewers or as a questionnaire to be filled in by the patient directly. Patients respond to each item in the questionnaire by choosing one of five possible responses: very often, fairly often, occasionally, hardly ever, and never. The computing of the overall and separate section scores can be done in different ways: by counting the number of positive responses, by calculating the rates (percentages) of the different responses given (within each section), thereby establishing which of the which of the five was most frequent, or instead by applying a series measures specially developed by the examiner to assess the importance of each response. With this latter method it is also possible to obtain a weighted analysis of the different sections, and therefore to understand which category of impairment impacts most on the patient's life.

The OHIP evaluation system was first used by Locker D [4] as part of a longitudinal epidemiological study of oral health. It emerged, from the analysis, that social factors were as important as clinical ones in revealing the impact of oral conditions on overall health. The OHIP was also found to be an efficient, reliable, valid, and generalizable instrument, equally applicable to both elderly and young subjects.

The OHIP was subsequently used to estimate the impact of facial pain and its consequences on QoL [5]. The OHIP lends itself to application not only in descriptive studies, but also in the clinical assessment of patients prior to treatment, as an aid in efforts to identify individuals who would most benefit from dental treatment, and as a clinical outcome measure.

Furthermore, the OHIP may also be used, together with clinical tools, as an "indicator of necessity," helping to identify of a subgroup of individuals, among those examined, whose clinical conditions have a significant impact on their daily life and who would therefore probably benefit more from a given dental treatment.

As we have seen, oral disorders can affect functional, social, and psychological well-being, and the availability of instruments (like the OHIP) for measuring this impact is enabling

dentists to apply the latest concepts of oral health care. Greater knowledge of the ways in which oral disorders and conditions affect the personal and social dimensions not only promotes greater understanding of the complexities of oral health, but also opens up the possibility of identifying interventions designed to minimize the consequences of this important group of diseases, and thus contribute to patients' well-being.

In the light of the above considerations, we developed an original research protocol on the impact of orofacial pain on QoL. We focused, in particular, on the presence of orofacial pain due to temporomandibular disorders (TMDs) [6].

This study was a cross-sectional case-control study.

A total of 124 new patients referred, with orofacial pain, to the Section of Prosthetic Dentistry and Temporomandibular Disorders of the University of Pavia were recruited as study subjects.

Pain was most frequently located in the temporomandibular joint (TMJ) (87.1%), and mainly related to chewing (71.0%); sizeable proportions of patients reported feeling pain in front of the ear (74.2%), tenderness of muscles at the side of the face (66.9%), and in and around the temples (62.1%) (Table 1).

In many cases, pain was triggered by performing a mouth opening movement (73.4%). More than half of the patients (57.3%) reported experiencing headaches quite frequently.

With regard to the intensity/severity of the pain, 43.5% of the study subjects described it as "irritating." When asked to rate it on a scale of

Table 1 Prevalence of pain in the last month

Symptoms	%
TMJ pain	87.1
Facial pain in front of the ear	74.2
Pain in an around the eyes	45.2
Pain on opening, widening the mouth	73.4
Shooting pain in the face or cheeks	27.4
TMJ pain when chewing	71.0
Pain in or around the temples	62.1
Tenderness of muscles at the side of the face	66.9
Frequent headache	57.3
TMJ sounds: clicks or popping/grating sounds	71.0

1–10, the proportion rating it 4–6 was the same as the proportion giving it a score of over 7 (42.75%).

Pain was a daily occurrence in 47.6% of the patients (Table 2).

The results showed that the greatest difficulties encountered by the patients in relation to their disorder were of a psychological nature: 56.4% of the sample claimed to be worried about their pathology and 54.8% said they were aware of it; 46.8% often felt tense, and 43.5% reported sleep disturbances due to the pain; 41.99% of patients said the pain could interfere with moments of relaxation during the day.

With regard to the practical difficulties reported by the patients, 49.2% had **difficulty chewing certain foods (especially foods with a rubbery texture that require prolonged chewing)** and 37.9% took **longer to finish a meal;** 39.5% had **difficulty eating some foods** and were thus often **forced to eliminate them from their diet** (35.5% of the patients) (Table 3).

The main functional issues were found to be linked to chewing: in particular, **difficulty chewing some foods** (to the point that these are often eliminated from the patients' usual diet), and **more protracted mealtimes**.

Most of the TMD patients **prepare food differently (eating a softer diet),** consider that their **choice of food is limited and** report **pain when eating**. Foods most often reported to be **difficult to eat** are **meat, apples, bread, toast, and toffees.** That could cause an **adequate intake of iron** [7].

Patients with more severe pain intensity are likely to **reduce their intake of dietary fiber** to decrease masticatory activity to avoid exacerbating facial pain. Low dietary fiber increases the **risk of constipation and bloating** [8].

Choosing foods that require less chewing can result in **weight loss or gain, loss of energy, digestive problems**, and/or **fatigue** [9].

Table 2 Characteristics of pain in the last month (% distribution)

	%
Severity	
Mild	9.7
Irritating	43.5
Moderately severe	23.4
Severe	16.1
Very severe	7.3
Likert scale severity score	
1–3	14.5
4–6	42.7
7–10	42.8
Frequency	
Daily	47.6
Between 2 and 4 times a month	25.0
Once a week or less	27.4
Duration	
1 h or less	53.2
Between 2 and 8 h or more	26.6
Between 9 and 12 h or more	20.2

Table 3 Questionnaire on the quality of life

	Fairly often/very often (%)	Occasionally (%)	Hardly ever/never (%)
Functional limitation			
Difficulty chewing some foods	49.2	22.6	27.4
Trouble pronouncing words	14.5	14.5	69.4
Taking longer to finish a meal	37.9	12.1	50.0
Psychological discomfort			
Feeling worried about the pain	56.4	19.4	24.2
Self-awareness	54.8	19.4	19.5
Feeling unhappy	23.4	18.5	55.7
Feeling tense because of the pain	46.8	22.6	29.0
Physical disability			
Speech is not clear	4.0	14.5	80.7
Some people cannot make out your words	4.0	11.3	83.9
Impossible to clean your teeth	12.1	6.4	80.7
You avoid eating some foods	35.5	17.7	45.2

(continued)

Table 3 (continued)

	Fairly often/very often (%)	Occasionally (%)	Hardly ever/never (%)
You have trouble doing jobs around the house	12.1	14.5	72.6
You have to interrupt your meals	16.9	16.9	65.3
You have difficulty eating some foods	39.5	14.5	46.0
Psychological disability			
The pain interferes with your sleep	43.5	20.2	36.3
You feel generally distressed	34.7	26.6	38.7
You find it hard to relax	41.9	25.0	32.3
You feel depressed	30.6	25.0	44.4
You struggle to concentrate	24.2	24.2	51.6
You feel embarrassed	14.5	17.7	66.1
Social disability			
You avoid going out with others	14.5	15.3	70.2
You are irritable with your partner	17.7	21.8	60.5
You have trouble getting on with others	10.5	15.3	74.2
You avoid eating with others	8.9	6.4	84.7
You avoid laughing in company	7.3	8.1	83.9
Handicap			
Can't enjoy yourself due to the pain	9.7	9.7	80.6
Less satisfied with life	12.9	14.5	72.6
Disabled to function	6.4	12.1	81.5
Disabled to work	13.7	16.9	69.4

2 Role of Diet and Nutrition in the TMD Management

Management of TMDs by conservative and reversible interventions has been shown to be both appropriate and successful.

Conservative treatment involves **counseling,** physical, and **cognitive behavior,** and **dietary therapies** [10].

Self-care, including resting, relaxation techniques, hot and/or cold packs, home remedies, and the **use of vitamins, nutritional supplements for pain** [11] or **Chinese herbs** [12], stretching or exercises, occlusal splint therapy, massage, manual therapy, and others should be considered as a first choice therapy for TMD pain because of their low risk of side effects. In the case of severe acute pain or chronic pain resulting from serious disorders, inflammation and/or degeneration pharmacotherapy, minimally invasive, and invasive procedures should be considered [13].

Counseling and self-management-based therapies are a conservative low-cost and beneficial treatment for treating TMD, with good results for the relief and control of TMD signs and symptoms by improving psychological domains and potentially reducing harmful behaviors [14].

This approach consists in:

- patient education about the multifactorial etiology of TMD and the rationale of cognitive-behavioral therapy
- guided reading with structured feedback, using participant-completed forms to explore the participant's understanding of and dentification with major themes, such as rationale for breathing and relaxation methods, TMD knowledge, communicating with health care providers, emotions, and bodily changes
- introduction to the role of stress and negative psychological states as potential factors in the exacerbation and maintenance of TMD pain
- self-monitoring of signs and symptoms in particular to detect parafunctional behaviors
- development of a *Personal TMD Management Plan*
- delivery of a brochure through which the clinician illustrates to the patient some simple, eas-

ily executable precautions, highlighting with a stroke of colored pen those most suitable for the individual case.

The treatment plan must be tailored to the individual patient and should seek to reduce or eliminate the pain, reduce the harmful loading, and ensure functional improvement and resumption of normal daily activities; it should also include stress control measures and, if necessary, **dietary re-education**.

Health care providers must devote time to understand the totality of the suffering of these patients and instead focus **only** on the medical aspects of treatment [9].

It could be useful the use of **a nutritional questionnaire and a food diary**.

The questionnaire must include questions as

- Has the condition of your jaw altered your diet?
- Is it painful to open your mouth to eat, bite, or chew?
- Are you avoiding any specific food groups, such as fresh fruits, fresh vegetables, whole-grain breads, or nuts, because of pain associated with TMD?
- Have you avoided going out for meals or eating with others because of TMD?
- How has your weight changed? [10]

The clinician must ask patients about food group intake, listing items such as fresh fruits, vegetables, protein-rich foods (meat, fish, poultry, nuts, and beans, vegetable protein sources like tofu), dairy products and fats and sugar-rich foods, drinks and vitamin, mineral, herbal, or other dietary supplements and comparing their responses to national standards. This simple assessment will provide some insight into unintentional weight change, dietary problems, and diet quality and can be used then to give the patient dietary guidance [15].

Clinicians should assess the level of symptom burden experienced by patients with TMD as it can impact patients' meals, snacks, and **socialization around mealtime** [10].

According to the cognitive-behavioral therapy model, environmental events do not impact mood and functioning directly, but are first mentally filtered and processed by the individual. If the individual is prone to distorted thinking (e.g., catastrophizing, overgeneralizing, or overpersonalizing), then the emotional impact of the event, as well as the coping response that follows, can become exaggerated, unhelpful or negative [16].

Cognitive therapy is based on the premise that modifying maladaptive thoughts results in changes in affect and behavior.

Behavior therapy is rooted in the theory that inner states (thoughts and feelings) are less important than the use of operant behavior change techniques to increase adaptive behavior through positive and negative reinforcement and to extinguish maladaptive behavior. Several behavioral techniques are applicable, including behavioral activation (getting patients moving again), graded exercise (initiating exercise and then slowly increasing activities), activity pacing (not overdoing it on days when patients feel good and remaining active on days when they feel bad), reducing pain behaviors (not reinforcing behaviors associated with secondary gain), sleep hygiene (identifying and then changing behaviors known to disrupt sleep), learning relaxation techniques (e.g., breathing, imagery, progressive muscle relaxation) [17], and **dietary re-education.**

It is very important to readdress the diet in order to avoid the **physical** (weight loss or gain, loss of energy, digestive problems, inadequate intake of iron, bloating, and constipation) and **psychological consequences** (socialization around mealtime) and to support a good general health [18].

It may be helpful to have in the multidisciplinary team a nutritionist/dietician to devise a **nutritious and palatable soft menu** and to find out what vitamins or other substances may be lacking in diet that could help support TMJ health and overall wellness [19].

3 Dietary Guidance for Patients with TMD

A **soft diet** is indicated. For people who are unable to tolerate a soft diet, a **pureed diet** may be better tolerated.

It is very important to eat **soft and easy to chew foods** such as soups, stews, steamed or cooked veggies, and protein smoothies.

Creamed soups are good soft diet foods, as is any other pureed or blended soup like chicken noodle.

"Soft bread buns/rolls" require more jaw movement to bite, chew, and swallow than foods such as popcorn kernels or chopped tomatoes, all of which have more dietary fiber than most soft forms of bread [15].

A balanced diet that includes cereals, legumes, vegetables, fish eggs, dairy products, meat, fruit, etc., must be maintained.

It is advisable to avoid prolonged chewing and excessive opening of the mouth.

3.1 Instructions and Advice for the Patient

- correct portions of food
- small bites
- slow and complete chewing
- relaxing meals
- light dinner
- mouth opening control
- no chewing gum
- no hard bread
- no whole apples (fruit must be peeled and cut, or as an alternative baked apples)
- no big sandwiches
- no hard meat
- no lettuce.

A *soft diet* is recommended for a 2-week period, following which a review determines whether the individual advances as tolerated to firmer and chewier consistency foods moving towards a *pain-free diet* [20].

A TMD Nutrition Guide Booklet guide is freely available online [21]. The guide includes a list of foods to include (like smooth yogurt, soft cheeses, vegetable soufflé, soft-cooked chicken or turkey) as well as to avoid (like nuts and seeds) and other helpful tips.

To **correct constipation**, it is recommended to increase fiber and drink more liquids (especially warm liquids). Good fiber sources include bran and other whole grains found in cereals, breads, and brown rice, beans, baked apples and pears, and prunes.

Prunes and prune juice are often touted as nature's remedy for constipation.

Good ideas and recipes in a **TMJ cookbook** [22].

If the patient has a neuropathic and neurovascular component, the **food composition or temperature** may exacerbate or play or role in triggering pain.

In trigeminal neuralgia, it may be related to **food temperature,** whereas in migraine it may be the presence of caffeine or tyramine in foods that trigger the pain [15].

From a treatment perspective, the identification of **algogenic substances** in foods helps to complete the multidisciplinary approach to TMDs.

The prevalence of TMD in the headache population is more than 50% and this prevalence tends to be higher in patients with combined migraine and tension-type headache [23].

Certain foods, beverages, and ingredients within foods may trigger attacks of headache and/or migraine in susceptible individuals. Elimination diets can prevent headaches in subgroups of persons with headache disorders [24].

The most common foods and beverages that have been self-reported to trigger migraine include chocolate, coffee, nuts, salami, alcohol, tomatoes, milk, citrus fruits, cheese, carbohydrates, leavened products, red wine [25], while the most frequent ingredients were caffeine, monosodium glutamate (MSG), artificial sweeteners, nitrites, gluten, and biogenic amines (e.g., histamine, tyramine, and phenylethylamine).

It is not reasonable for persons with headache to avoid all know dietary triggers, as individuals may only be susceptible to a small number of foods or beverages. If a food, beverage, or ingredient is identified as a trigger, it should be avoided to reduce the frequency of headache. The triggers could be identified by simple observation if the association is strong or through the use of a food diary if it is less obvious [26].

There are a number of diets that could be employed for persons with headache. The three diets with the most promise include the **high omega-3/low omega-6** [27, 28] and low fat diets as well as the elimination diet of IgG positive foods.

Linoleic acid is the predominant omega-6 polyunsaturated fatty acid (PUFA) that promotes inflammation. The omega-3 PUFAs are alpha-linolenic acid, which comes from plants such as flax, and docosahexaenoic acid (DHA) and eicosapentaenoic acid (EPA), which come from fish, organic free-range eggs, and grass-fed beef. Omega-3 PUFAs promote anti-inflammatory pathways.

The choice of a specific diet may in part depend on comorbid medical conditions as well as the type of migraine encountered by the patient.

Ketogenic diets might also be considered in some patients [29]. Based on overlap between mechanisms postulated to underlie pain and inflammation, and mechanisms postulated to underlie therapeutic effects of ketogenic diets, recent studies have explored the ability for ketogenic diets to reduce pain.

Some minerals like **magnesium** plays a role in reducing headaches and muscle spasms [19].

Orofacial pain of an inflammatory origin such as arthrogenous TMD, it is plausible that antioxidant status may play a role in the pathophysiology of the condition. **Vitamins C, D, and E, soy, carotenoids,** and **an array of dietary flavonoids** have been shown to have antioxidant properties and anti-hyperalgesic effects [15].

Here a list of anti-inflammatory foods: all leafy green vegetables, avocados, yams, berries, nuts and seeds, lentils and beans, quinoa, buckwheat, whole grains and pro-inflammatory foods: sugar, bread, pastries, processed cereals, white rice, white potatoes, deep fried foods, and red meat [30].

Increased parathyroid hormone levels in response to vitamin D deficiency seem to be more prominent in patients with TMDs. These data suggest that, in patients with TMDs, **vitamin D** deficiency should be investigated and corrected [31].

Glucosamine supplements have been a topic of interest in several human clinical trials, as they are usually well tolerated and might present therapeutic effects that alleviate joint disease symptoms, but their use in the management of TMJ osteoarthritis to address pain and maximum mouth opening (MMO) restriction are still controversial [32].

Both glucosamine sulfate and ibuprofen seem to reduce the pain levels in patients with temporomandibular degenerative joint disease [33].

Among dietary constituents, substances that contain polyphenol compounds (resveratrol, chlorogenic acids, catechin, and genistein), carotenoids (lutein), and fatty acids (docosahexaenoic acid [DHA] and decanoic acid [DA]) could affect peripheral and central nociceptive neuronal pathways, including the trigeminal pain pathway [34].

For **Chinese Medicine** most TMJ causes involve a yin-blood vacuity failing to nourish the sinews (or muscles) of the jaw. In this case, proper diet is extremely important as well as supplementation with Chinese herbs which nourish the blood.

The combination of Chinese and western medicines could be a very effective combination for the treatment of TMJ.

According to Chinese medicine, foods to eat are whole grains, especially barley, millet and sweet rice, beans and bean product, such as tofu and tempeh, sea vegetables, such as arame, nori, kombu, and wakame [35].

There are several herbs (that can also be used in teas, cooking, and topically) that can alleviate TMJ pain by reducing anxiety, stress, inflammation, and help get better sleep [36].

Ginger has been used for over 5000 years in cooking and other medicinal uses. Traditionally, ginger has been used for nausea, pain, and inflammation.

Ginger can be used in teas, cooking, baking, and of course for healing purposes.

Turmeric is another herb that has been used in cooking and for its medicinal uses. The main active constituent is curcumin which gives turmeric its yellow color. Another, constituent is, borneol oil it helps reduce inflammation and

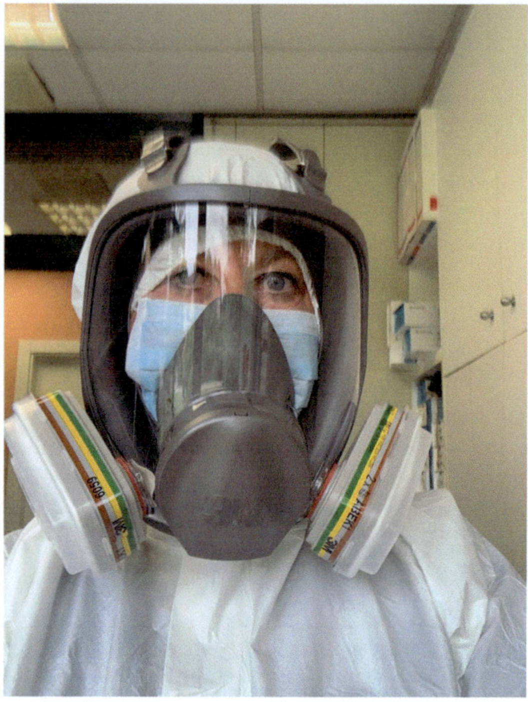

Fig. 1 Marzia segu working in COVID-19 conditions

valepotriates is an analgesic. Turmeric can be used in tea, cooking, baking, topically and for gum pain.

The next herbs are **valerian, kava, and lavender**. These herbs are known to reducing stress, anxiety and improve sleep. Individuals who suffer from TMJ can benefit by incorporating these in teas, foods, and baths.

The dietary program must be tailored [37] (Fig. 1).

References

1. Haketa T, Kino K, Sugisaki M, et al. Difficulty of food intake in patients with temporomandibular disorders. Int J Prosthodont. 2006;19(3):266–70.
2. Bitiniene D, Zamaliauskiene R, Kubilius R, Leketas M, Gailius T, Smirnovaite K. Quality of life in patients with temporomandibular disorders. A systematic review. Stomatologija. 2018;20(1):3–9.
3. Slade GD, Spencer AJ. Development and evaluation of the oral health impact profile. Commun Dent Health. 1994;11(1):3–11.
4. Locker D. The burden of oral disorders in a population of older adults. Commun Dent Health. 1992;9(2):109–24.
5. Murray H, Locker D, Mock D, Tenenbaum HC. Pain and the quality of life in patients referred to a craniofacial pain unit. J Orofac Pain. 1996;10(4):316–23.
6. Segù M, Lobbia S, Canale C, Collesano V. Quality of life in patients with temporomandibular disorders. Minerva Stomatol. 2003;52(6):279–87.
7. Irving J, Wood GD, Hackett AF. Does temporomandibular disorder pain dysfunction syndrome affect dietary intake? Dent Update. 1999;26(9):405–7.
8. Raphael KG, Marbach JJ, Touger-Decker R. Dietary fiber intake in patients with myofascial face pain. J Orofac Pain. 2002;16(1):39–47.
9. Safour W, Hovey R. A phenomenologic study about the dietary habits and digestive complications for people living with temporomandibular joint disorder. J Oral Facial Pain Headache. 2019;3(4):377–88.
10. Nasri-Heir C, Epstein JB, Touger-Decker R, Benoliel R. What should we tell patients with painful temporomandibular disorders about what to eat? J Am Dent Assoc. 2016;147(8):667–71.
11. Riley JL III, Myers CD, Currie TP, et al. Self-care behaviors associated with myofascial temporomandibular disorder pain. J Orofac Pain. 2007;21(3):194–202.
12. Ritenbaugh C, Hammerschlag R, Dworkin SF, et al. Comparative effectiveness of traditional Chinese medicine and psychosocial care in the treatment of temporomandibular disorders-associated chronic facial pain. J Pain. 2012;13(11):1075–89.
13. Wieckiewicz M, Boening K, Wiland P, Shiau YY, Paradowska-Stolarz A. Reported concepts for the treatment modalities and pain management of temporomandibular disorders. J Headache Pain. 2015;16:106.
14. Manfredini D. A better definition of counselling strategies is needed to define effectiveness in temporomandibular disorders management. Evid Based Dent. 2013;14(4):118–9.
15. Durham J, Touger-Decker R, Nixdorf DR, Rigassio-Radler D, Moynihan P. Oro-facial pain and nutrition: a forgotten relationship? J Oral Rehabil. 2015;42(1):75–80.
16. Molton IR, Grahamb C, Stoelba BL, Jensena MP. Current psychological approaches to the management of chronic pain. Curr Opin Anaesthesiol. 2007;20(5):485–9.
17. Hassett AL, Gevirtz RN. Nonpharmacologic treatment for fibromyalgia: patient education, cognitive-behavioral therapy, relaxation techniques, and complementary and alternative medicine. Rheum Dis Clin N Am. 2009;35(2):393–407.
18. Levrini L. La dieta del sorriso. Mangiare bene per la salute della bocca. Milan: Mondadori Electa; 2016.
19. Michaud-Bonyadi J, Bonyadi D. Your roadmap to TMJ health: how to navigate your way through TMJ disorder with a comprehensive approach to healing.

Toronto, ON: Hasmark Publishing International; 2018.

20. Durham J, Al-Baghdadi M, Baad-Hansen L, et al. Self-management programmes in temporomandibular disorders: results from an international Delphi process. J Oral Rehabil. 2016;43(12):929–36.

21. The Temporomandibular Joint Association (TMJA). TMD nutrition and you. n.d.. http://www.tmj.org/Publications.

22. Coffield B. You can conquer TMJ ideas and recipes. Wickenburg, AZ: Moonlight Mesas Associates; 2007.

23. Ballegaard V, Thede-Schmidt-Hansen P, Svensson P, Jensen R. Are headache and temporomandibular disorders related? A blinded study. Cephalalgia. 2008;28(8):832–41.

24. Martin VT, Vij B. Diet and Headache: Part 1. Headache. 2016;56(9):1543–52.

25. Razeghi Jahromi S, Ghorbani Z, Martelletti P, Lampl C, Togha M. School of Advanced Studies of the European Headache Federation (EHF-SAS). Association of diet and headache. J Headache Pain. 2019;20(1):106.

26. Martin VT, Vij B. Diet and Headache: Part 2. Headache. 2016;56(9):1553–62.

27. Ramsden CE, Mann JD, Faurot KR, et al. Low omega-6 vs. low omega-6 plus high omega-3 dietary intervention for chronic daily headache: protocol for a randomized clinical trial. Trials. 2011;12:97.

28. Ramsden CE, Zamora D, Makriyannis A, Wood JT, Mann JD, Faurot KR. Diet-induced changes in n-3- and n-6-derived endocannabinoids and reductions in headache pain and psychological distress. J Pain. 2015;6(8):707–16.

29. Masino SA, Ruskin DN. Ketogenic diets and pain. J Child Neurol. 2013;28(8):993–1001.

30. Tick H. Nutrition and pain. Phys Med Rehabil Clin N Am. 2015;26(2):309–20.

31. Demir CY, Ersoz ME. Biochemical changes associated with temporomandibular disorders. J Int Med Res. 2019;47(2):765–71.

32. Melo G, Casett E, Stuginski-Barbosa J, et al. Effects of glucosamine supplements on painful temporomandibular joint osteoarthritis: A systematic review. J Oral Rehabil. 2018;45(5):414–22.

33. Thie NM, Prasad NG, Major PW. Evaluation of glucosamine sulfate compared to ibuprofen for the treatment of temporomandibular joint osteoarthritis: a randomized double blind controlled 3 month clinical trial. J Rheumatol. 2001;28(6):1347–55.

34. Takeda M, Shimazu Y. Modulatory mechanism underlying how dietary constituents attenuate orofacial pain. J Oral Sci. 2020;62:140. https://doi.org/10.2334/josnusd.19-0224.

35. Monte T. The complete guide to natural healing. New York, NY: TarcherPerigee; 1997.

36. Gonzalez J. Using healing herbs to relieve TMJ pain. n.d.. https://www.livingeatinghealthy.com/blog/using-healing-herbs-to-relieve-tmj-pain/.

37. Deodato F, Di Stanislao C, Giorgetti R. L'Articolazione Temporo-Mandibolare. I DTM secondo valutazione tradizionale e integrata con Medicine non Convenzionali. Rozzano, MI: Divisione Universitaria - CEA Casa Editrice Ambrosiana Zanichelli Editore; 2005.

Prevention Strategy: A Practical Protocol for Elderly Patients

Alexander Mersel and Gil Zvi Eisenberg

1 Sub-Chapter A: The Challenge

1.1 Prevention Strategy for the Not to Be Neglected Elderly Patients, a Practical Approach

Elderly population growth has increased in the last decades dramatically causing a demographic change affecting the dental clientele spectrum. We treat older patients in age and in numbers. These patients demand good quality dentistry regarding treatment plans and aesthetic outcome [1].

They demand better living quality and are willing to pay for it.

With the ability to provide such demands coms a responsibility to maintain good oral health and avoid pitfalls and failure.

This article will try to establish a practical protocol for elderly patients follow-up and check-up.

1.2 The First Foundation in Establishing a Good Protocol Should Be Starting in the Treatment Plane

The treatment plane should foresee the future of the patient.

When considering the health prognosis of an elderly patient one must understand that the prognosis will eventually deteriorate, by this we mean physically, manually, and psychologically.

All these parameters will reduce and so will the ability of the elderly patient to maintain a simple home protocol of self-dental hygiene. This will eventually affect the prognosis and the survival of the treatment.

Having said that an understanding of these facts should be achieved with the patient and family/guardian/children/sibling (A.K.A companions).

The right match of the right plan should be agreed upon after specifying and warning of all.

What could go wrong in time as a cause of aging and health deterioration?

The patient and companions should reach an understanding of the importance of follow-up meetings and treatment in order to prevent deterioration or failure.

Special emphasis should be in planning and explaining of alternatives plans and alternatives when a tooth, crown, bridge or prosthesis fail.

A. Mersel
Community Dentistry Hadassah School of Dental Medicine, University of Jerusalem, Jerusalem, Israel
e-mail: mersal@netvision.net.il

G. Z. Eisenberg (✉)
Assuta Hospital, Tel-Aviv, Israel

Understanding of the end result of alternative treatment upon failure must be achieved by patient and companions and documented.

Understanding of the increasing role of companions in future contacts scheduling and appearing to appointments is crucial.

Contact protocol with patient and companions should be established and documented.

Example timetable should be presented and understand.

1.3 The Second Foundation of the Treatment Is the Follow-Up Protocol

1.3.1 Follow-Up Protocol Should Contain

Visual Examination and Carries Detection Dental carries increases with age due to decreased immunological response to external bacteria, coronal, and root carries are more active in older population but root carries have double prevalence [2].

Special emphasis should be held on root carries detection and treatment.

The significance of caries elimination on teeth survival is great and easily understood by patient and companions. It has a very high response by the patient by means of motivation and acceptance of help if needed in keeping of daily oral hygiene procedures and also in treatment by dentist, oral hygienist, and fluoride appliance [3–5].

X-ray examination (if needed) should also help in carries detection and the evaluation of existing restorations prognosis.

Periodontal Examination Prior to treatment plan, periodontal chart, and evaluation of teeth stability. These will be the base line and referendum for the follow-up inspections and reevaluation in the future. So (if needed) the same or part of the periodontal evaluation is needed as a part of the protocol.

Experimental gingivitis studies showed faster supra gingival plaque development in older patients than in young ones [6].

The immune system is not as active as it used to be. Smaller amount of bacteria could cause bigger damage periodontal speaking.

We need to assess the risk to reduce infections and improve self-sustainability [7]. If that could not be obtained we should re-consider our plane.

Salivary Glands Function and Mucus Quality With aging a reduction of saliva and a change of saliva quality and pH is known.

With increasing age the reserve capacity for production saliva by salivary glands is diminished causing salivary hypofunction [8].

Salivary hypofunction increases the chance for caries, candidiasis, and denture discomfort [8].

In addition there are more than 700 medications known as abele to decrees and change saliva quality, all these lead to dry mouth, bad taste, bad breath, I will refer all these as Xerostomia [9].

But most of all could increase caries (especially root caries) and cause mucosal irritations. Special care should be made on oral cancer detection. Effort should be made to document and reevaluate medications changes and follow-up for salivary glands function and mucus quality, if these occur maybe a consult should be carrying out whit the patient's physician in order to intervene before it affects the patient's quality of life and dental prognosis [10].

Oral Cancer It increases its occurrence with age. It could be detected in various areas in the mouth but is commonly detected under removable prostheses and near badly shaped restorations or broken or sharp angled teeth causing mucosal irritation. Special efforts and examinations should be made especially under removable dentures and oral mucosa in order to detect and eliminate the cause. It is crucial to send a biopsy, get a pathological analysis and carry a close follow-up.

Candidiasis Oral candidiasis has a higher detection in patients with removal prostheses and xerostomia. Also as mentioned before there is a decrease of immune system ability. All of these may cause oral candidiasis.

Detection and treatment by means of increasing oral hygiene, denture cleaning, and drug therapy is simple but need to be done and carried by a follow-up.

Those measures are all that is needed but sometimes a complete technical chemical denture cleaning is needed as well.

Angular Cheilitis It is commonly connected with candidiasis and denture stomatitis. Sometimes it is caused by a wrong and decreased V.D. of the prostheses or rehab. But sometimes on some neuromuscular problems involving orbicularis oris. The cause should be detected, evaluated, and treated. Topically & solving the cause.

2 The Third Foundation Is Documentation

All means should be considered: meeting dates, patient appearance, state of health and mind, so for companions.

These should be kept and documented in an orderly manner: charts, records and evaluations, X-rays, and photographic documentations and imaging, study models, old used provisional, written and verbal consults with other clinicians. Written and verbal agreements with patient and companions. Future follow-up schedules and their target.

3 The Fourth and Last Is the Clinicians Point of View Judgment and State of Mind

Dental treatment for the elderly is eventually by long-run perspective a "losing ware."

We may wine some battles but in the long run no one could beat time, wear out, aging physical and mental fatigue.

The possibility that treatment failure due to causes not depending on doctor or patient's ability is big, sometimes inevitable.

It takes a very strong and determent clinician to stand up for that task and role. It is very easy to fall into frustration. And so dental treatment for elderly is not for everyone, "It takes a Special breed."

A word of advice, try personalizing as much as you can to your own world, try thinking of him or her as a member of your family. It is not only the sympathy but the more important. Accountability needed for the job.

3.1 Conclusion

In the above I tried giving a short and simple view of what I as a simple G.P. see as a treatment and follow-up protocol for the elderly patient. I would like to hope that sharing my point of view helped.

4 Sub-Chapter B: The Challenge

4.1 Education

Obviously the ultimate gate for a good prevention approach cannot ignore the role of Education.

In the first part we demonstrated the important task of the Dentist. There is a strong obligation to set up a comprehensive Education and Training for the Dental Profession.

Education is divided into several different categories:

1. Basic Education.
   The duration of forming an average dentist, DDR, DMD is (for the formation of future Dentists, DDR, or DMD) usually 5–6 years (study) with clinical training and examination before obtaining a State License.

   The Institutions delivering the Diplomas are; Dental Schools Or Dental Faculty within Universities or Private Organizations.

Their syllabus is based on the majority of Oral and Dental Issues.

On the undergraduate level very little attention is paid for Gerodontics or for Special/Handicapped patients [11].

2. Advanced education or Post-graduate formation is devoted for Practitioners looking for a better comprehension (in) or a Specialty.

At the term of devoted study cycle the Dentist obtain a Specialist diploma. The Diploma Gerodontology diploma is actually not frequent in The Dental Institutions [12].

3. Continuing Education.

The FDI/World Dental Organization have underlined the fact that Continuing Education is an ethical obligation [13].

This issue is now running in European Main countries, nevertheless there are different systems and education plans running.

On the one hand, the Universities or Dental Faculties and, on the other hand, the Professional organizations (Associations or Chambers).

In one or 2 years, participating a number of courses, Congresses, Seminars, and other recognized events a Dentist will receive an official Attestation [14].

Unfortunately when actually checking their curriculum, scrutinize the Programs seldom Place any interest in Geriatric Dentistry or Special Treatments issues (Oral Health 2000).

4.2 Aims and Means of Continuing Education

A long life Continuing Education (C.Ed) started several decades ago. But the major question is who will be the main target group for that C.ed. (Fig. 1). If the challenge is Global Oral Health,

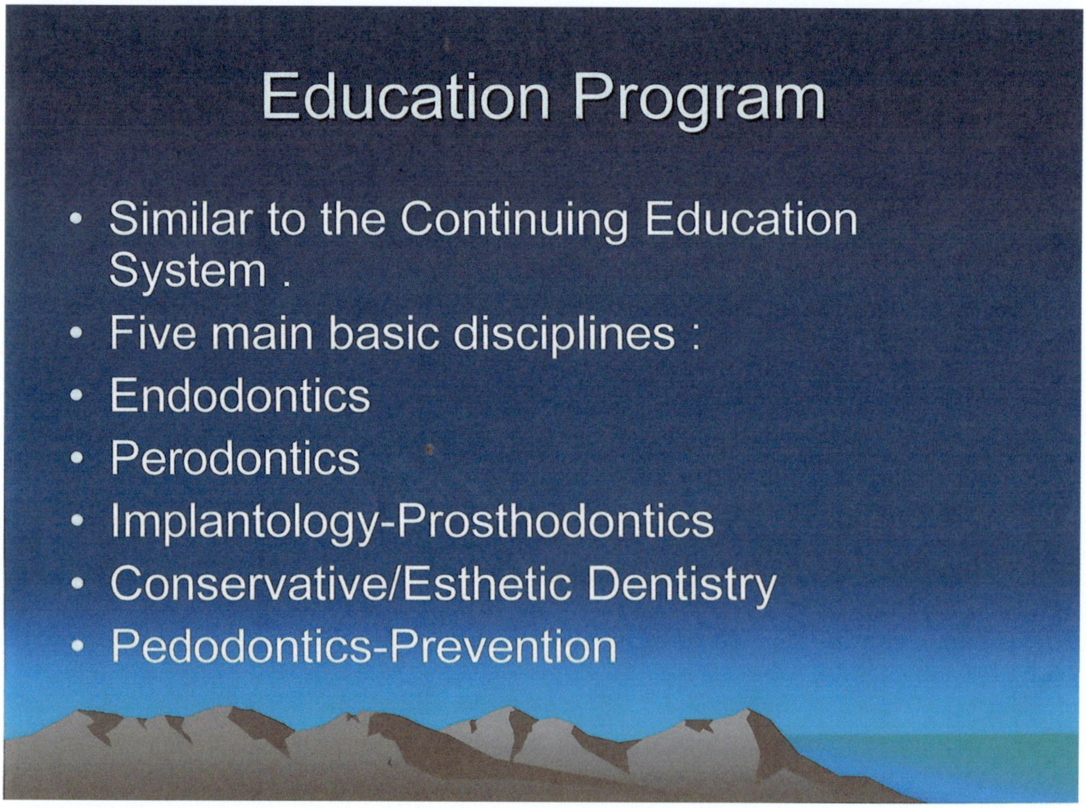

Fig. 1 The most important disciplines chosen by the dentists; there is no prevention

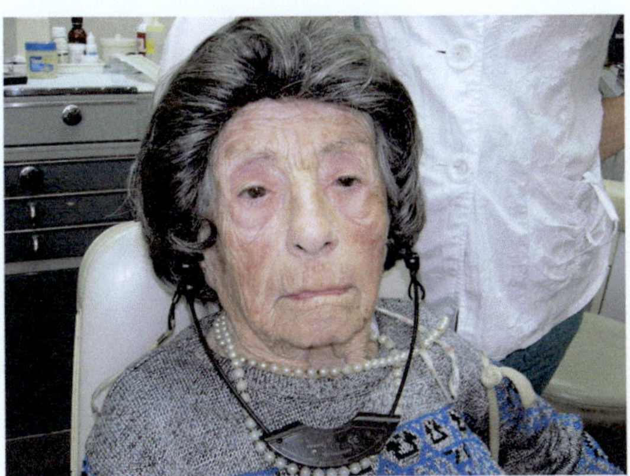

Fig. 2 A 100-year aged patient utilizing Dental Hygienist Prevention Program

Prevention is a key issue; General Practitioners (GP) should be in front of this action. Looking for effective Prevention protocol they have to act as Oral Health officers.

Therefore, the C.Ed Program is not the concern of high level specialists and not for undergraduate students.

It should focus on the G.P., (but also for) the Dental Hygienist and the Dental Assistants (Fig. 2).

The question of the responsibility of this formation is crucial. Obviously there are three main partners.

1. The Public Health Institutions as official representing the Public Health policy.
2. The University and the Dental Faculties (as delegating) focusing on their education systems.
3. The Dental National Associations, gathering a majority of Dental Practitioners and could act as a in general a good center of coordination. The Dental Chambers and the Liberal Educations Centers (Colleges, Scientific Associations, and Scientific Revues) are all within this peer group.
4. The last but not least; the Dental Partners (the Industry).

The industry's influence us in different levels:

In our experience our partner influence is at different level critical:

By the choice of focusing on the Items: Implantology, Cad-Cam, Perio-Implantology, and Esthetic Dentistry.

By the choice of speakers, very high level Personalities or and often commercial minded Lecturers (Fig. 3).

By the determination of the Lecture—time, place, and schedule (early in the morning or late at the end of the session).

All of the above mentioned shifts the peer groups focus and neglects the much needed focus on Gerodontics issues.

A. Mersel and G. Z. Eisenberg

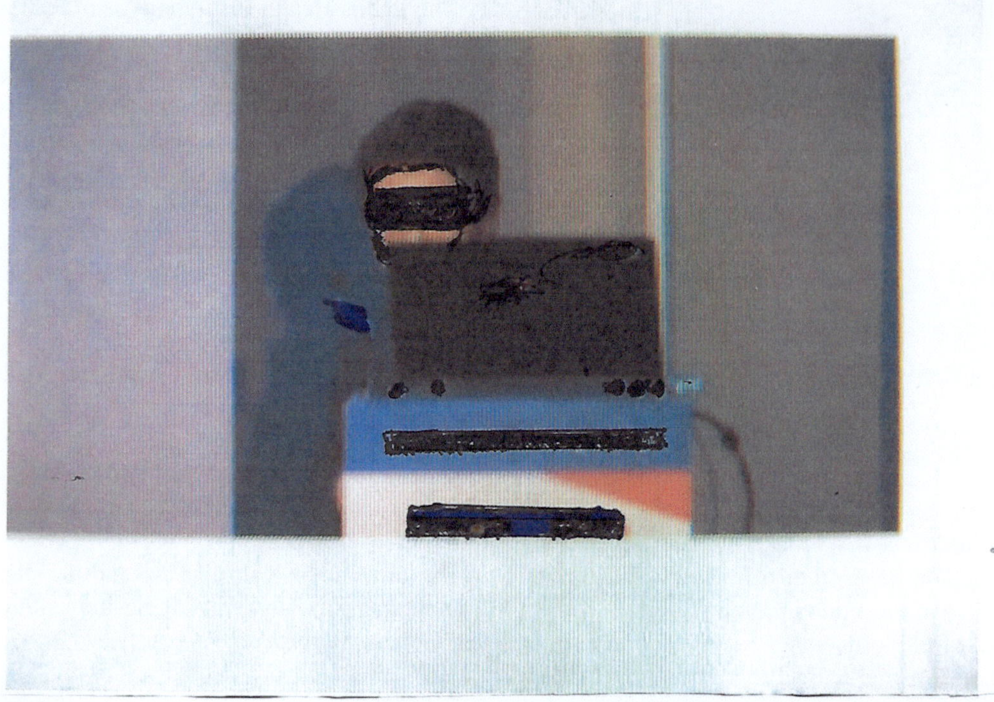

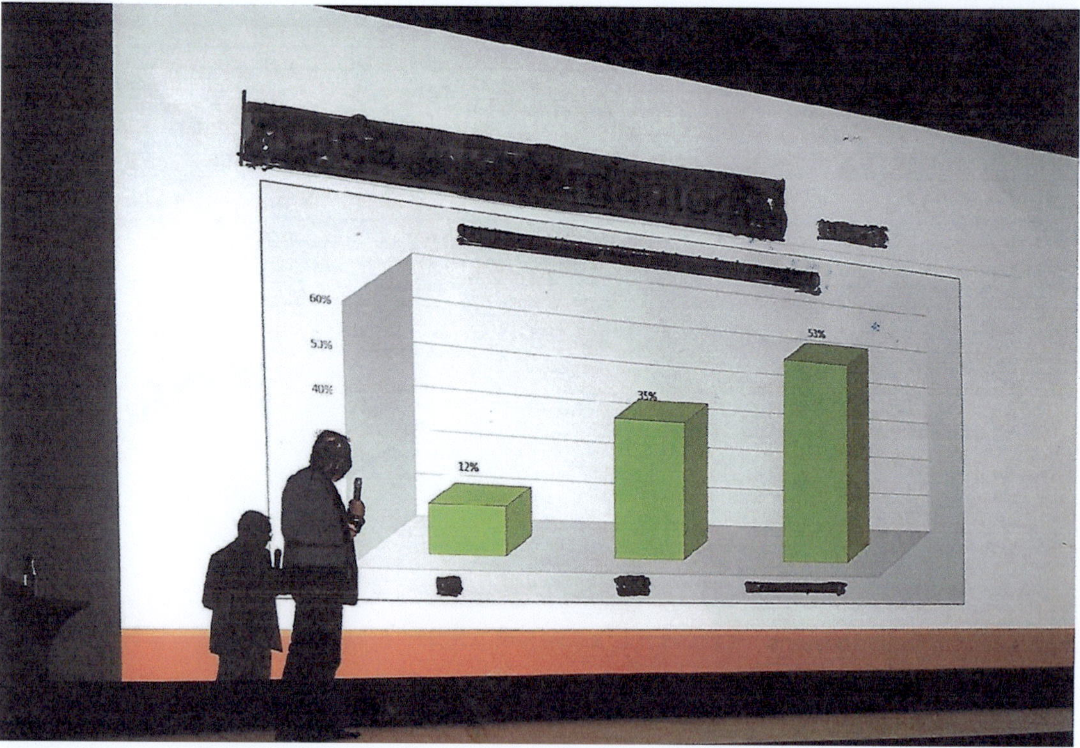

Fig. 3 Unappropriate position of the speaker; behind the laptop or on the platform

5 Discussion

If Prevention is our Priority, there are fundamental facts to be clarified. In the actual dentistry approach a side the classic dental treatments concepts, CED system should strongly focus on clinical applications as result of the last dental and scientific advances (ERO UN 2011).

The fact is that the CED, voluntary or compulsory, does not give us any indication of the satisfaction of the Dentists Participating at those events regarding Gerodontics education, research and development.

In general after the Lecture an evaluation is asked or made by a questionnaire. Since there is no obligation to fulfil the Questionnaire, the survey is of little value and cannot be utilized.

A new innovation is: We could easily facilitate the questionnaire by taking advantage of the cell phone technology in order to receive the Dentists opinion, but as long that this is based on voluntary attitudes there is no certitude on the results.

Therefore a new system was set up in order to collect the attitudes forward the Education Program. During several years this approach was successfully promoted (Evaluation Georgia) (Fig. 4).

5.1 Results

Report on the data's that are mainly presented: Tables 1 and 2. Very surprising data was gathered in a survey about the Satisfaction of the Continuing Education Program in Jerusalem [15].

5.1.1 Satisfaction

A: 63% for the Lecturer.

B: 47% for the Presentation.

C: 57% for the Topic.

D: 69% for the Facilities.

E: 45% for the expectations.

We witness the disruption between the appreciation of the Lecturer and the final satisfaction [16].

Therefore, when looking for a good transmission of our prevention message and a strong motivation of the participants a serious evaluation is necessary.

This lead to the Problem of The Speakers [16].

5.2 Guidelines for the Speakers

We perfectly understand that a poor Speaker can deliver a bad presentation. Nobody is born with a talent of a Speaker. If each Lecture is like an

Evaluation after the lecture : Satisfaction				
	Presentation	Application	Question Answers	Facilities
2010 Batumi	39 %	60 %	68 %	51 %
2011 Tbilisi	59 %	36 %	52 %	68 %
2012 Tbilisi	77 %	65 %	67 %	78 %

Fig. 4 Evaluation by the audience about the satisfaction of the presentation

Opera, an appropriate training is necessary, unfortunately we often are frustrated by a disaster session (Fig. 1).

Since the Prevention topic is relatively new in Cont.Educ, we should pay a special attention to this topic.

5.2.1　In Educating the Educators [17]

There are basic and simple guidelines.

1. The Position. The Speaker should not be isolated from the Forum and hidden behind the desk and the Laptop (Fig. 2).
2. The microphone should also be mobile giving freedom for two hands and without a cumbersome wire. A head neck micro is recommended.
3. The number of slides must be adapted to the importance of the topic, if the minimalistic time of each slide is about 2 min, in 1 h the speaker cannot exceed 30 slides per hour. Caution if there is tables or slides with several subjects/photos the number of slides will drop down to 35/40 (Fig. 3).
4. The contact with the audience is compulsory.
5. During the Lecture the Speaker has an obligation to look.

    On at the audience (the public), the best is if he is able to go down from the Platform.

The voice volume, the clarity of the pronunciation, the variation of the intonation are the "sine qua non" to avoid a monotonic speech.

A good speaker will deliver his Topic with real motivation [18].

5.3　Looking for the Future

The Profession has advocated a strategic preventive protocol in order to achieve a preventive goal: "20 teeth for the eighties." This target is only possible by an evidence based approach and a realistic low-cost treatment Plane [19].

The FDI/World Dental Organization had already stated that: "Prevention is better than restoration." [20].

Unfortunately the last terrifying COVID-19 epidemic catastrophe will certainly carry important socio-economic changes.

Because financial problems, we expect a rise in dental non-attendance among low-income patients (it's expect, a dental non-attendance among low-income patients). Therefore, intensive Prevention is absolutely necessary in order to maintain a minimal Oral Health [21].

5.4　Conclusion

We have to develop an Educational Program focused on Oral Health and Prevention.

We must advocate a Continuing Education system for the Oral Health workforces for the training and the treatment of the neglected patients. A side this approach it is recommended to open a dialogue with all the professional parties promoting a real popular Prevention Dynamics.

References

1. Berkey D, Meckstroth R, Berg R. An aging world: facing the challenges for dentistry. Int Dent J. 2001;51(3):177–264.
2. Hand JS, Hunt RJ, Beck JD. Incidence of coronal and root caries in an older adult population. J Public Health Dent. 1988;48(1):14–9.
3. Thomson WM. Dental caries experience in older people over time: what can the large cohort studies tell us? Br Dent J. 2004;196(2):89–92.
4. Luan W, Baelum V, Fejerskov O, Chen X. Ten year incidence of dental caries in dult and elderly Chinese. Caries Res. 2000;34(3):205–13.
5. Drake C, Beck J, Lawrence H, Koch G. Three-year coronal caries incidence & risk factors in North Carolina elderly. Caries Res. 1997;31(1):1–7.
6. Holm-Pendersen P, Agerbaek N, Theilade E. Experimental gingivitis in young and elderly individuals. J Clin Periodontol. 1975;2(1):14–24.
7. Kiyak HA, Persson RE, Persson GR. Influences on the perception & responses to periodontal disease among older adults. Periodontol. 1998;16(1):34–43.
8. Turner MD, Ship JA. Dry mouth & its effects on the oral health of elderly people. J Am Dent Assoc. 2007;138:S15–20.

9. Shetty S, Bhowmick S, Castelino R, Babu S. Drug induced xerostomia in elderly individuals: an institutional study. Contemp Clin Dent. 2012;3(2):173.

10. Wiener RC, Wu B, Crout R, Wiener M. Hyposalivation & Xerostomia in dentate older adults. J Am Dent Assoc. 2011;141(3):279–84.

11. Naimie Z, Ahmad NA, Shoaib L, Safii S. Curriculum for special care dentistry: are we there yet? J Int Oral Health. 2020;12(1):1–7.

12. Mersel A. An adapted continuing education program in Gerodontics : the actual challenge. J Global Oral Health. 2018;1(1):1–4.

13. Kossioni AE, et al. An expert opinion from the European College of Gerodontology and the European Geriatric Medicine Society: European Policy Recommendations on oral health in older adults. J Am Geriatr Soc. 2018;66(3):609–13.

14. Mersel A. Speaker guidelines lecturing in continuing education. J Israel Dent Assoc. 2015;32(2):32–6.

15. Mersel A, Tayeb I. Continuing education: evaluation of the dentists satisfaction in two countries. SF Dent Oral Res. 2018;J.2(1):1–4.

16. Mersel A. Speaker Guidelines in Continuing Education. J Israel Dent Assoc. 2015;32(2):32–5.

17. Mersel A, Margvelashvili V, Margvelashvili M. Evaluation in continuing education. Dental Asia. 2013;7(8):20–2.

18. Mersel A, Baruch M, Tayeb I, Mann J, Zini A. Dentist's satisfaction of continuing education: survey among dentists in Jerusalem. J Israel Dent Assoc. 2017;34(1):53–66.

19. Thomason JM. Treatment for the older person minimum standards or minimal care. Eur J Prosthodont Res Dent. 2005;15(4):140–6.

20. Oral health for an ageing population. OHAP task force FDI. 2019. www.fdiworldental.org.

21. Schimmei M. Preventive strategies in geriatric dental medicine. J Oral Health Prevent Dentis. 2016;14(4):291–2.

22. Marchini L, et al. Geriatric Dentistry education and context in a selection of countries in 5 continents. Spec Care Dent. 2018;1281:1–10.